GREAT LIVES IN BRIEF
A Series of Biographies

ACCURACY
CLARITY
MULTUM
IN PARVO

HENRY FORD by Roger Burlingame
MAHATMA GANDHI by Vincent Sheean
ALEXANDER DUMAS by André Maurois
HANS CHRISTIAN ANDERSEN by Rumer Godden
CHARLES DARWIN by Ruth Moore
JULIUS CAESAR by Alfred Duggan
JOHN L. HILL by Samuel Hopkins
ELIZABETH I by Donald Barr Chidsey
NAPOLEON III by Albert Guerard
CHARLES STUART by James Thomas Flexner
NAPOLEON I by Albert Guerard
ROBERT E. LEE by Earl Schenck Miers
GARIBALDI by Denis Mack Smith
WOODROW WILSON by John A. Garraty
LOUIS PASTEUR by Pasteur Vallery-Radot
ST. FRANCIS OF ASSISI by E. M. Almedingen

These are
BORZOI BOOKS
Published by Alfred A. Knopf
in New York

GREAT LIVES IN BRIEF
A Series of Biographies

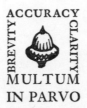

ACCURACY
BREVITY CLARITY
MULTUM
IN PARVO

These are
BORZOI BOOKS
Published by ALFRED A. KNOPF
in New York

MAHATMA GANDHI

Mahatma Gandhi

A GREAT LIFE IN BRIEF

BY

Vincent Sheean

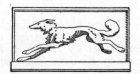

New York   ALFRED A. KNOPF   1970

L. C. catalog card number: 54-7222

THIS IS A BORZOI BOOK,
PUBLISHED BY ALFRED A. KNOPF, INC.

PUBLISHED JANUARY 24, 1954

REPRINTED THREE TIMES

FIFTH PRINTING, APRIL 1970

CONTENTS

CONTENTS

MAHATMA GANDHI

CHAPTER ONE

BEFORE THE BATTLE

GANDHI's existence from the beginning of the present century was subjected to a more rigorous public attention than any other known to us. Everything he said and did was recorded and made public immediately. His pulse-beat and his bowel movements were precisely noted. He could not condone a sin without assuming its guilt. Once when he permitted a doctor to chloroform a hopelessly sick calf, the whole of India was in turmoil. When he was unable to sleep, millions did not sleep; when he fasted, millions fasted; his slow, gentle words were cut into wax and disseminated by radio to half a continent several times a day. He had the unparalleled misfortune to become a public saint in the twentieth century, canonized alive in the glare of flashlights and the relentless gaze of cameras. Only the most resolute attention to his immediate tasks, toilsome and endless, enabled him to ignore the world's fantasies and keep on going. He had to cultivate, deliberately and with immense difficulty, a patience that was not originally in his nature, so as to endure the environment of his greatness. "The woes of Mahatmas," he said wryly, "are known to Mahatmas alone."

Yet the myth arose and was a true myth, changing the behavior of whole populations, altering the course of history and the fate of empire. There is no other case known to us in which every fact is known and yet their sum amounts to an unknown. We cannot satisfactorily explain the phenomenon of Gandhi. The efforts made by *Pravda*

and by the *Philosophical Review* in Moscow, during the
year that followed his death, were the most absurd manifestations of epigonic Marxomania that even those peri-
odicals have exhibited. There is far more truth in a phrase
Lord Halifax once used in talking of Gandhi to me: "He
was a good little man." The gentle and kindly Viceroy
knew the temper of his antagonist: they understood each
other.

Goodness might be, of course, the key. My own guess
is that the Mahatma thought it was. The only claim he
ever made for himself was to have lived the greater part
of his life (almost fifty years) in the most literal and exact
effort to obey the teachings of the *Bhagavad-Gita*, to
which he assimilated the Sermon on the Mount. This
was essentially an ethical preoccupation, not metaphysi-
cal; he was not a philosopher. He wanted to be good, to
live the good life, and goodness was for him very much
associated and almost identical with innocence. ("I eat
only innocent food," he said to me.) The regaining of
lost innocence may seem a hopeless endeavor, and certainly the Mahatma himself was troubled by a sense of
failure in some respects. He was never fully reconciled
to the idea of drinking goat's milk, though it had become
a physical necessity. He had to overcome anger at times,
impatience at other times; the subjugation of lust was an
agony, a victory as difficult as the Lord Buddha's subjugation of the wild elephant. Whatever his imperfections
as they appeared in his own eyes, it is not easy to imagine
any human being whose ethical nature was more system-
atically controlled than his toward the end of his life, or
more harmoniously adjusted to the instinctive good.

Goodness, just the same, cannot explain the power of
the Gandhi myth. It is beyond dispute that his person-

ality commanded even when he least desired to command. An identity of opposites haunts his entire story: it
is just when he was most humble that he was most powerful. To the very end this Hegelian interaction obtained,
for it was by his death that he achieved the ultimate purpose of his life. His death was, indeed, a singular fulfillment, coming at a time when he felt his own people drift-
ing away from him, summoning them once more (and all
the world besides) to one moment of salutary awe.

To what, then, are we to assign the phenomenon, to
what shall we attribute the magic?

We come at last to the mystical explanation as the only
one that fits the case. It fits because it presupposes the unknown and beyond that the unknowable. The grace of
God, as Christians call it, is the only tenable hypothesis.
Otherwise the life of Gandhi, even though fully proved
in every fact, has no historic intelligibility. There must
have been in his discrete genius a general component, a
pulse from the common pulse, a force both vertical and
horizontal in its thrust, so that he could communicate
more than others and hear a voice that others do not hear.
He did actually hear an "inner voice" throughout the
greater part of his life (just as Socrates did), and though
he was an exceedingly practical man who never discussed
mysteries if he could help it, there is no doubt in my own
mind that the essence of his effective being, effective, that
is, upon mankind, was and always will be a mystery.

2

He was born in one of those very small princely states
which used to make a patchwork in the west of India,
above Bombay. His own state was Porbandar, of which
his father was Prime Minister as his grandfather had been

before that. His family belonged to the merchant caste (Bania) and to the Vaishnava side of the Hindu religion. The Vaishnava, worshipping Vishnu in various aspects, though not exclusively, have been increasingly numerous in India since the sixteenth century, and various doctrines of sin, redemption, and divine grace have arisen among them—not in response to any Christian influence, so far as is known, but by internal development. These ideas do not find expression in the other great school of Hinduism, which worships chiefly Shiva.

In Porbandar, where the Gandhi family lived, there were a good many members of the Jaina sect, those who refuse to take any life under any circumstances. Jains were frequent visitors and lifelong friends of the family, and it is no doubt quite true that they all felt the influence of Jaina beliefs. Even so, Gandhi claimed to be an orthodox Hindu throughout his long life, and although many of his interpretations (as to caste and the like) disturbed the pundits, Hinduism is large enough to contain almost any variation, and his claim to orthodoxy was never seriously contested.

His parents were devout indeed, and he always attributed the steadfastness of his behavior, in such matters as vows and disciplines, to the power of examples always before him in his childhood. Most of all his mother and his nurse, pious Hindu women of their rather strict sect, exerted this power and were never forgotten. His mother, for example, sometimes fasted when the sun did not shine, in obedience to some vow taken perhaps years before. The children used to watch anxiousy on cloudy days for the first ray of sunshine, so as to run shouting to her that she could now eat.

Mohandas Karamchand Gandhi, the future Mahatma,

was born at Porbandar on October 2, 1869. He was the youngest son of Karamchand Gandhi, known as Kaba, who was Prime Minister at various times in no less than three of those little Kathiawar states—Porbandar, Rajkot, and Vankaner. Kaba Gandhi's father and one of his brothers had held similar positions. They were not quite such exalted positions as the words might indicate, for these were small states, and none of the family accumulated much wealth. But Kaba Gandhi was, by his son's recollection, an extremely able man in the practical sense, dealing with all the intricate clan questions and disputes that arose in his jurisdiction. He was a great temple-goer and took to reading the *Gita* toward the end of his life, repeating some verses every day in the family worship. This, too, must have had a formative effect on young Gandhi's mind.

But on the whole the boy was not remarkable; according to his own testimony, at any rate, he showed no great aptitude for study. He was extremely shy through his early years and afraid of companions; he tells us that he used to run to and from school to avoid having to talk to anybody. One episode of his childhood seems to have made a great impression: it was a performance he saw by a traveling dramatic company of the play *Harishchandra*, based on a great story in the *Mahabharata* epic. It narrates the sufferings of a king of old who sacrificed everything for the truth and went through almost endless ordeals before his redemption. Only a few days before his death, Gandhi told me this story himself at considerable length; once a thing like that entered his consciousness it could not be dislodged. As a child he used to act out *Harishchandra* to himself, as he said, "times without number." The idea of the truth as supreme good was thus early implanted, and seems to have grown as naturally in him as a tree or a flower. It was to become, in time, a central and almost a single idea governing every region of his thought.

He was married, by family arrangement, at the age of thirteen. His delight in his bride, Kasturbai, was extreme, and in later years he regarded this premature sensuality with sorrow and shame. It may have contributed to his strong views on child marriage, which he regarded in his maturity as one of the great evils of India. At that time it not only was legal, but was valued among Hindus as a salutary protection against the world. In the time and place these arranged matches between children previously unknown to each other were universal, and it has often been remarked that happy marriages were usually the result. It was so, in any case, with Gandhi, and although his conscience in later years troubled him greatly, he found Kasturbai the solace of his life so long as she lived.

The boy Gandhi was lustful, possessive, and, as he tells us, unreasonably jealous. The customs of the period allowed him to meet Kasturbai only at night during the half year that she spent in the Gandhi household; the other half of the year she spent with her parents. He wanted to teach her everything he knew, since she was illiterate, but "lustful love," as he called it, gave him no time to do so, and Kasturbai remained without instruction beyond simple letters in the local language, Gujarati. His regrets and self-condemnation are quite explicit in his autobiography.

He, of course, continued into high school, regardless of his marriage: "Only in our present Hindu society," he said, "do studies and marriage go thus hand in hand." He had his difficulties with study, but after his fourteenth year seems to have made much better progress, actually winning a prize or two along the way. In his own account of these years he makes much of a regrettable episode involving an older boy who was addicted to eating meat and drinking wine in secret.

The older boy, originally a friend of Gandhi's brother, held that India's troubles would be solved if the Hindus took to eating meat. He used to quote a bit of doggerel to this effect:

> Behold the mighty Englishman:
> He rules the Indian small,
> Because, being a meat-eater,
> He is five cubits tall.

The older boy could reinforce his argument by being, himself, much stronger than Gandhi, able to run and jump and exhibit his muscles. Young Gandhi resolved to try meat-eating out of a mixture of motives—to make himself stronger; to see Indians grow stronger; to get meat-eating started as a sort of "reform." On the first occasion the two boys repaired to a lonely spot by the river and attacked a piece of goat's meat. It made Gandhi sick, and that night he had nightmares of a goat kicking in his stomach. Later on, for about a year, more delicate preparations of meat were made from time to time by the older friend, and Gandhi actually learned to like them. The feasts were few and far between, he says, because the boys had no money. He finally gave up meat-eating, not because he regarded it as wrong in itself, but because it inevitably led him into telling lies to his pious parents.

The same older friend also took young Gandhi to a

brothel, but there his shyness protected him ("God in His infinite mercy," he says, "protected me against myself"). He was never in his life unfaithful to Kasturbai.

These misdemeanors culminated in a fling at cigarette-smoking, for which Gandhi pilfered some coppers from home and also a chip of gold off his elder brother's arm-band. This time Gandhi's conscience revolted at last. He wrote out a complete confession and submitted it to his father with a request to be punished. This was accompanied by a pledge never to steal anything again. His father's suffering and tears remained in his memory ever afterwards.

Such boyish misdeeds may seem slight indeed in Western eyes. They had enormous importance in a pious Vaishnava family. The Jaina influence, as has been said, made the Gandhi family even more rigid in observance than some others might have been, and the eating of flesh was regarded by them all with abhorrence. The cigarette-smoking was not in itself of any great importance, but to steal coppers and tell lies in order to smoke was much worse.

The final sin, which he calls "my double shame," occurred when Kaba Gandhi died. Young Gandhi had been his father's nurse, rubbing his legs and attending on him in his illness. At the same time he was much preoccupied with "lustful love," as Kasturbai was in the house. One night he went from his father's sickbed to his own bed-room and woke Kasturbai up. She was then pregnant, and his very keen remorse was partly due to this. While he was with Kasturbai a servant knocked on the door to tell him that his father was dead.

The child that was born to Kasturbai lived only three or four days. Gandhi's sorrow over the whole episode was deep and remained with him even when he came to write of it many years later.

3

Hindu students seldom went overseas in the 1880's. To do so meant, as a rule, expulsion from one's caste, for association with foreigners, eating foreign food, and enduring various and complicated contaminations were unavoidable on such journeys. This is all thoroughly out of date now, and seems to a modern Indian as remote as the Middle Ages to us, but it was still the state of opinion in Gandhi's youth. Those who had gone to England and returned to India were thought to be lost to their own religion. They were "as bad as foreigners" because they wore foreign clothing, indecent because it outlined the elements of the human body, and because they frequently ate foreign food. The point of view of that day is lost now. Hardly anybody in India can remember when trousers were thought indecent; nobody objects nowadays to the smoking of cigars or cigarettes; even meat-eating is condoned on a wide scale, although most Indians are still vegetarians. In the 1880's the Hindus who went abroad and came back to their profitable enterprises as barristers, doctors, or merchants (and the barristers predominated) were looked upon as renegades and, in fact, as contaminated.

The notion of contamination is still not lost in India. When Gandhi was young it was vital in its ghostlike way—as vital as any ghost can be. The shadow of an untouchable falling across any part of the body of a caste Hindu was a contamination and required of that caste Hindu a process of ceremonial purification. This is still true with some elderly and devout people. A caste Hindu could accept milk from an untouchable, but not water. In the very lowest castes the process of discrimination obtained, so that even among the untouchables one sub-division could perform one task but not another. The almost incredible divisions of labor into which the original caste system proliferated may have been due in part to the excessive population or the general poverty, but it resulted in a complicated series of discriminations that have since been gradually and naturally disappearing.

Gandhi was not afraid of any of this. When his family's old friend and adviser Mavji Dave, a Brahmin who had been a lifelong friend of the dead father, advised study in England, the young Gandhi leaped at the prospect. His first idea was that he might study medicine, but the Brahmin adviser was against it. Medicine was contrary to the old religion—that is, Western medicine, with its insistence on dissection of the body's organs—but, more important, a medical doctor could never be prime minister of a state. The Brahmin adviser wanted the young Gandhi to be a prime minister, like his father, uncle, and grandfather, and for this position a knowledge of the law was most important. The earlier Gandhis had been almost illiterate, but had ruled because they had known their clans and castes and personalities. Young Gandhi was to succeed to their functions by means of the new weapons to be obtained in England, by admission to the bar. As he was eighteen and still continuing his studies (whereas his brothers had forsaken them), the family adviser thought the youngest son should go to England and study law.

So he did. It was not easy. The objections to vanquish were many—from the clan and caste, from the uncle, from the mother. The mother, a simple and devout woman, was not afraid of the ocean in particular, or of the far places, but she dreaded what she had heard of women, wine, and meat-eating in foreign lands. When she had the firm vow of her son to abstain from any of these habits, she reluctantly and sorrowfully consented. He took his vows before a Jaina monk who had once been a Hindu of his own caste, and this satisfied the mother's objections. The vows were never violated.

But on his arrival in Bombay he ran into more caste difficulties, and was in fact, after some debate, solemnly read out of his own caste. (It was the *Modh Bania*, a fraction of the *Bania* fraction of the *Vaishya*.) No member of his caste had ever gone overseas before, and in a solemn meeting it was declared that he would be contaminated. He accepted this without difficulty, and, what is more surprising, so did his elder brother. He remained outcaste to the end, though as a "holy man" he was (by Indian definitions) exempt from all caste rules or regulations. He never again observed any of the caste rules, such as the wearing and manipulation of the "sacred thread," a symbolical cord, or the various shavings and not-shavings which were part of the ritual. In his own mind he was truly outcaste, and chose to remain so.

He was only eighteen, a shy and eager Hindu boy with ears stuck out almost at right angles from his head, when he sailed from Bombay on September 4, 1889. He had new European clothing, purchased through the offices of his brother and friends. The necktie, which was to become a source of pleasure to him in London, was then a torture. He was acutely conscious of his short jacket and trousers. Shoes were unpleasant. But he was equipped for the great journey and alive with anxiety to learn, to acquire the instruments of victory.

All instruction in India above the first four classes of
elementary school was then, as now, conducted in English. Thus Gandhi had an acquaintance with the English
language before he ever went to England. But it was a
school-language, not the language of the mother or the
market, and it did not come naturally to him. On the ship
he had difficulty understanding what anybody, even the
stewards, said to him. He was afraid of violating his vows
against wine, women, and meat and consequently ate all
his meals in his cabin, chiefly from food he had brought
with him. The poor boy knew nothing of the knife or
fork, and was so shy that he was afraid of speaking to any
fellow passenger. Moreover, he had saved his best clothing, which was white flannels, for his landing at South-
ampton (having worn black all the way to England)
and consequently landed in the grisly English autumn
weather most unsuitably dressed. This was his chief anxiety for two days, until he could obtain his scanty baggage. He wept at night for a long time, strange and alone,
uncertain of every step, fearful of violating his vows un-
wittingly or of committing some other Indian sin in an
English climate.

The first problem was, of course, food. It does not
matter so much any more to Indian students. It did not
matter much even then to a great many of them. They
ate what the country provided and got used to it. But
Gandhi had taken the vegetarian vow, which he was determined to observe or die. He could not eat the sodden,
savorless substances that constituted the English idea of
vegetables. He has recorded that in the early weeks he
almost starved. Oatmeal porridge in the morning was a
help, but at other meals it was difficult to know what to
do. The Indian student friends among whom he found

himself—who had found a boarding-house for him—
were incensed. They had no difficulty eating meat and
thought Gandhi both foolish and obstinate in his insistence upon his vegetarian vow. From one boarding-house
to another he took his weary way, never getting his fill,
until one day he hit upon a vegetarian restaurant in Far-
ingdon Street. "God had come to my aid," he said. He
found in that restaurant, where he at last had a hearty
meal, a copy of a book called *A Plea for Vegetarianism*,
which he bought for a shilling and took with him. He
read it over and over and it converted him—that is, converted him from being a vegetarian by inheritance and by
vows taken to the mother, a matter of religion and tradition, into a vegetarian convinced of the rightness of his
cause. As usual in his long life, he had found something
to support him in what he already was and already believed. He had found "authority." He could now be a
vegetarian on a theoretical basis.

It is curious and, of course, funny that Mahatma Gandhi was forever in search of "authority" for his few,
simple, and sovereign ideas. Once he said to an inter-
viewer: "Everything I have to say is as old as the hills."
This was true, except that the circumstances and surroundings of the saying made a great difference. And yet,
old as his ideas were, he sometimes took many long years
to find out that something he intimately felt and believed,
with all the power of his intense being, was felt and believed by others or had been felt and believed by others
before him. This kind of discovery, recurrent not often
(because the ideas were few) but powerfully, made
every great turning-point of his life. His vegetarianism
was as natural, as inborn, as anything could be in a human
being, and yet a few books and pamphlets by English

proselytists (known, of course, as "cranks") gave him the strength to see that what he was could be justified rationally. In this respect the entire life of Gandhi is a story of becoming what he already was, of becoming himself. He was it, but he required these external buttresses to assure himself that he was or might be right. His humility, overwhelming at the end, must have been innate or he could not have relied so heavily upon these accidental aids from the beginning. It was so in all the subsequent discoveries, with Tolstoy or Ruskin or Thoreau—they each in turn came to support with "authority" that which he already passionately believed and had already acted upon to the limit of his powers. It was so even with the *Gita* and the New Testament, which incised themselves into his soul by words corresponding to the realities already existent there.

The vegetarian battle occupied a good deal of his time in London. His Indian friends thought it was improper and embarrassing of him to insist on food contrary to the surrounding customs. He tried, in his tenderhearted way, to make it up to them by being as elegant as possible, as conformable to English customs as his purse and temperament would allow: he bought evening clothes, took dancing lessons, tried to learn the violin, and made in general an attempt to "play the English gentleman," as he said. He seems to have spent several months in these preoccupations, endeavoring to make up by social graces for the obstinacy with which he clung to his vows to his mother. In the end he surrendered all that, suddenly and completely, to devote himself to his studies for the bar.

The photographs of Gandhi taken at this age (and published by him) are extremely funny—the little Hindu boy with ears at right angles, the piercing eyes and meager face, the stiff high collar and pomaded hair. He was prob-ably conscious even then of how funny the whole enter-prise was. There never was any time in his life when he could not and did not laugh at himself. Indeed, laughter, of a gentle and innocent kind, usually at his own expense, was a necessity to him. Even two days before his death he made little jokes to me, and his oldest and most de-voted friends, such as Sarojini Naidu and Jawaharlal Nehru, had as many funny things as solemn ones to tell of him. Mrs. Naidu's stories show that throughout their long relationship the salutary virtue of the laugh sustained them both, even through anguished times.

4

Gandhi's three years in England were fruitful in many ways. After his first agonies were over he learned how to enjoy life and work in an English climate and on English terms. Vegetarianism was a help in unexpected ways; he joined the Vegetarian Society, became a member of its executive committee, and had his first experience in or-ganization, though shyness made him unable to speak at meetings. On the one occasion when he felt impelled to try, somebody else had to read his paper for him. And yet with the vegetarians he formed friendships and made acquaintances, just as he did among the students.

His first experiments with clothing, food, and Eng-lish life suddenly lost their interest for him when he de-cided that he had come to London to study and had done little in that direction. Admission to the bar was easy enough: not much study was required, the examinations were simple, and the "call to the bar" was automatic if the student had "kept terms" (twelve of them), equiva-lent to about three years. Gandhi therefore made up his mind to work for the London matriculation examination, and spent a whole year on it. It was given every six months, and he had only five left to prepare for the first one, in which he failed because of insufficient Latin. He took the examinations again six months later with (except Latin) different subjects. The second time he passed in all. The episode, with its unnecessary hard work—unnecessary in the sense that nobody expected him to undertake it—and with its excellent results, useful to him in many respects later on, was characteristic of Gandhi even at that age.

Also it was in England that he read for the first time both the *Bhagavad-Gita* and the New Testament. Two Englishmen, theosophists and brothers, introduced him to the *Gita*. Another Englishman, whom he met in a vegetarian boarding-house, induced him to read the Bible. He found it impossible to get through the Old Testament, but the New Testament, coming so soon after his first acquaintance with the *Gita*, profoundly impressed him—"went straight to my heart," he says.

It seems a little odd that Gandhi should not have known the *Gita* in either Sanskrit or his native Gujarati, for it must have been familiar to his father in both languages. He read it first with his English theosophist friends in the English metrical translation of Sir Edwin Arnold (*The Song Celestial*), which remained to the end his favorite translation of the great poem. The revelation must have been, at the very beginning, supremely personal: he found in the *Gita* exactly what he needed for the expression of what he felt in the recesses of his being, however obscurely, to be the truth. The advice of the Lord Shri Krishna to the hero Arjuna on the eve of the great battle is, indeed, a kind of crystallization of

Gandhi's characteristic beliefs, those upon which his own life struggle was based, and it is difficult to suppose that he could have done what he did without it; but the receptivity of his nature, its instinctive and immediate response, indicates that the teaching of the *Gita* was in him already in some unformed, some latent state. He was only twenty at the time, but already his own effort was directed toward the suppression of desire, appetite, and "attachment" in a larger purpose. The *Gita* reinforced his nature and gradually became the law of his life. Eventually he was to take it as a sort of book of practical rules, a specific directive.

The New Testament, in particular the Sermon on the Mount, had a similar effect, less powerful perhaps because it was Christian rather than Hindu; but during the years to come it was to entwine itself into all of Gandhi's thought and become in effect a kind of extension of, or variation upon, the *Gita*. The earliest evidence of this influence, which he remembered with delight long years afterwards, was the great verse on "resist not evil."

These discoveries were not followed by any great preoccupation with religious thought, for by this time the young man was actively studying for the bar. Most students in those days hardly bothered to read the textbooks. Instead they studied, and mostly in the last few weeks, notes on previous examinations, thus setting their wits or their luck against the probabilities. Gandhi determined to read everything; and for Roman law he elected to read Justinian in Latin. Thus he was busy enough at all times, and, with his increasing emphasis on economy in diet and living, he could not have found it very difficult to keep the vows he had made to his mother. And no doubt, in spite of that lack of general reading which he later de-

plored, he was actually better prepared for the bar examination, more thoroughly grounded in the texts and authorities, than most of his English fellow students.

He passed his examinations, was called to the bar on
June 10, 1891, enrolled in the High Court on the 11th,
and sailed for India the next day.

The formative value of these years was great, exter-
nally as well as within himself. Thus it was an advantage
later on that he had actually studied Roman law and read
Justinian in Latin; he had done it only as hard work and
discipline and because he would be forced to remember
it better that way; yet, as it turned out, much of what he
did in South Africa in the years to come depended on
this knowledge of Roman law, on which Dutch law was
based. He was mortally shy, and great difficulties were
in store for him on that score, but he was intellectually
prepared for his coming work much better than he sus-
pected, and in fact much better than he ever admitted
later on. He remembered himself as a very limited and
shy young man with no knowledge of the world, yet
there must have been few of his age at the bar who had
really read, *really* studied, the basic texts of their profession.

5

In India for the next two years Gandhi was, by his
own account, a failure. He began his return home, on the
very first day, by learning that his mother had died in his
absence. His brother, who carried on the family correspondence and sent him the money to keep going in London, had thought it best to conceal this event, which to
Gandhi was a blow even worse than the death of his
father.

And, of course, his knowledge of English and Roman law, however thorough, did not make up for a total ignorance of Indian law. He had to start an entire new set of studies, meanwhile establishing himself as a barrister and living in the manner, and with the expenses, which were thought suitable to that estate. He tried.

In the very first case he obtained as a barrister in Bombay, Gandhi found himself unable to utter a word. He got up to cross-examine the plaintiff's witnesses and, facing the court, came near to fainting. He sat down and told his client's agent that he would have to give up the case, that another barrister should be engaged. It was his first and last appearance as a barrister in India.

Bombay, with high prices and living standards, was not for a barrister who was too shy to speak in court. Gandhi went home to Rajkot to earn a living by making out briefs for other lawyers, drafting applications, memorials, and the like. This period of his life was not happy, and his first acquaintance with the arrogance of a British officer—one he had known in England—did not help much. The habit of giving commissions here and there, of using influence, intrigue, and petty politics in carrying out the business of the law, was also repugnant to him, so that he was more than ready when a chance came to leave it all behind him.

The chance came from South Africa, where a considerable number of Indians was already established in business and a larger number, as Gandhi was to learn, had been brought in as contract labor.

The offer came to Gandhi's devoted elder brother, quite possibly as the result of some discreet scout work on the brother's part. A Moslem Indian firm called Dada Abdullah and Co. had a claim for some forty thousand

pounds which had been dragging through the South
African courts for years. The proposal was that young
Gandhi should go to South Africa for a year as a guest
of the firm, with all expenses paid, to advise on the
further conduct of this lawsuit, as well as on the firm's
correspondence and other matters. He was to make himself useful, more or less as an employee of the firm, and
would receive one hundred and five pounds in cash and
all expenses.

It was not the most brilliant offer in the world, but
Gandhi was making no headway in India. The idea of
going to South Africa, of which he knew nothing, appealed to him, even though he would have to leave his
family behind. Obviously Gandhi, who was then twenty-
four, could have had no idea that South Africa would in
the next period of his existence alter everything for him,
form his destiny in a new direction, and return him to
India, eventually, as a national hero and a "Mahatma."
Such an extraordinary evolution through two decades
seems rather startling even now, when all of its elements
have receded into history. The South African epic, and
with it the creation of the Mahatma, must have been a
long series of surprises both to the hero of the story and
to those around him. For at no time can we discern anything like a plan: the plan was evoked by circumstance,
and only looks like a plan when it is all over. As Gandhi
lived through it, step by step, it was much more like an
endless sequence of improvisations, all reaching toward a
plan, of course, and becoming one in retrospect: one that
was to be used on a larger scale—indeed, on the largest
—when the time was ready for it.

CHAPTER TWO

DISCOVERY IN SOUTH AFRICA

THE SOUTH AFRICA to which Gandhi went in 1893 conformed in outline to the Union of today, with significant differences. That is, it consisted of four units: Natal, the Orange Free State, the Transvaal, and the Cape Colony, of which only the last bore a distinctly English imprint. At that time the Orange Free State and the Transvaal were Boer Republics, with Dutch (in the African version) as their official language. Natal, with a very mixed population, had been annexed to the British crown in 1845 after some lively vicissitudes, but except for Durban, its chief city, it had no great number of English settlers or businessmen. The restless spirits of many adventurers were abroad, and it was a brawling time, as we learn from many other sources (not Gandhi). The great men of the period were Paul Kruger in the Transvaal (President), F. W. Reitz in the Orange Free State (President), and Cecil Rhodes in the Cape (Prime Minister). John Henry Brand, the wise and conciliatory President of the Orange Free State, had died four years before. Men of sense and acumen were all aware that some day the destiny of the wonderful region would demand its union for the simplest geographic and economic reasons, yet racial and linguistic antipathies were still so powerful that reason could scarcely be heard. The Boers seem to have hated the English with a passion very difficult to comprehend, a passion more intense than that aroused in (for example) the Irish under conditions not dissimilar in some respects. The Boers felt that all South

Africa was theirs and that the English were arrogant inter-
lopers. They had made the "Great Trek" with all their
belongings, including vast herds of cattle, when the English took over the Cape Colony. They did the same thing
on a smaller scale when the English annexed Natal. Now
they were bitterly entrenched in the Transvaal and the
Orange Free State, herdsmen and farmers and horsemen,
a race of Dutch cowboys landlocked in their domain and
resentful of any intruder. An explosion was inevitable
because the discovery of gold and of diamonds some years
before had brought a flood of greedy men into the Boer
Republics from all over the earth. These *uitlanders*, as
the Boers called them, were hated and discriminated
against by every means possible and had no votes or
voices in government. It was clearly the desire of Paul
Kruger, President of the Transvaal, to get rid of them if
he could, as it was his deepest regret that gold and diamonds existed in his territory.

These conditions provided a most unstable atmosphere
throughout South Africa, except, perhaps, in the Cape
itself. It was only two years until Rhodes, that buccaneer
of genius, was to stimulate all antagonisms by organizing
the Jameson Raid against the Boers; there can be little
doubt that he wanted what he eventually got, which was
war. The government in London was, as always through
the nineteenth century, far more cautious or reluctant
than its agents and representatives in the field. But the
whole of South Africa in 1893 must have been seething
with hatreds, resentments, rapacities, and ambitions which
made it anything but an abode of peace, even for the
Europeans. Small wonder, then, that those who were not
European lived in terror.

We have grown familiar in our own day with the

South African nomenclature in regard to races. "European" means any person of pure white race. "Native" means an African. "Colored" means a person of mixed race. "Asiatic" means a person whose racial origins can be traced to Asia; in practice this means Indians, there being few others of Asian origin there. Any and all of these four divisions may be native to the country, but the divisions still remain fixed. That is so today; but when Gandhi went there, the oak was still, so to speak, an acorn, large numbers of the "European" and "Asiatic" persons were relatively newcomers, and the "colored" (mixed) population, now so important, was then much smaller.

If we did not already know Gandhi's character we might be surprised to perceive, in his autobiography, letters, interviews, and other utterances through the years, how little he noticed of all this. As an intelligent and educated young man he must have been aware of it, but with the extraordinary concentrated impetus of his whole nature, he lived with and for the Indians. Two decades in South Africa left him more Indian than before; indeed, it was in South Africa that he learned Sanskrit (as much as he ever learned it), that he memorized the *Gita*, renounced the world, and became the Mahatma. He went there in a stiff collar and a frock coat, determined to travel first-class and live in a style becoming a barrister of the Inner Temple. He left South Africa determined to revert to homespun and the life of the Indian poor.

And it is odd, indeed, that the struggles between Europeans, or of the Europeans against the natives of the country, affected him so little. There was something bestowed, endowed, or, if you like, stricken, about Gandhi: he behaved like a specific instrument of a specific purpose from

the beginning to the end of his life. In Africa he lived for
the Indians and thought only of the Indians. The wild
struggle of the others concerned him only as it affected
the lives of his own people. He passed through that turmoil without having had, so far as one can tell, one single
truly political idea, and without formulating any general
notion of the South African future except as it might re-
late to the Indian inhabitants. His activity, so admirable
in its purity and astounding in its results, thus bore little
relation to the general life of the society in which it took
place. Perhaps for this very reason the victory he obtained
in the end was static rather than progressive: it was great,
but went no farther, and since he left Africa in 1914 the
Indians have gained nothing beyond what he gained for
them. Their plight at the present moment, though different in every circumstance, is identical in *kind* with that
in which Gandhi found them in 1893.

Of this plight he knew nothing at all when he sailed
from Bombay. It took six weeks for the ship to get to
Durban, with stops at various ports on the way. The ship
was crowded, and Gandhi could get a berth only in the
captain's cabin, by that officer's kindness. The captain
taught him chess, and the fellow passengers were friendly.
It was not until he got off the ship at Durban, to be met
by Abdullah Sheth, his new employer, that he noticed a
difference in the manner of Europeans toward Indians.
He was to learn a great deal in a short time—a very few
days, in fact.

Abdullah Sheth, a rich but illiterate Mohammedan
merchant, was at first uncertain how to deal with Gandhi.
Nobody like Gandhi—that is, no educated Indian who
was a London barrister wearing English clothes—had
ever appeared in Natal before. The Indian merchants in

South Africa were prosperous, but had made their own way in a new country by cunning and acumen, without other advantages; they cared little for "hygiene and sanitation," those lifelong preoccupations of Gandhi's; they knew hardly any English; their *esprit de corps* did not exist except when they were collectively under some menace; they accepted without much resentment a great many disabilities and indignities from the European overlords. Most of the merchants were Moslems, with a sprinkling of Parsees and Christians; a good many of the clerks and bookkeepers were Hindus. The Moslems tended to call themselves "Arabs," and the Parsees called themselves "Persians" in a vain attempt to escape from the stigma of being Indian at all. Indians were known among the Europeans as "coolies," whatever their occupation or race or religion, and Gandhi—the only Indian barrister in South Africa—soon became known as "the coolie barrister."

All this he learned quickly, in considerable consternation. Abdullah Sheth was his tutor and seems to have warmed to the stranger after a few days. Gandhi learned, for example, that these well-to-do Indian merchants and their staffs had little or nothing to do with the much larger population of Indian workers who had been brought to South Africa under "indenture"—that is, as contract laborers for a period of five years. The workers were mostly from southern India, speaking Tamil or Telugu, and the merchants were from the north, speaking one or another of the northern languages. The workers, moreover, were all illiterate, a depressed community with, practically speaking, no rights. As soon as Gandhi became aware of their existence, they were much in his thoughts, but by the nature of things he had no

contact with them for some time: his task was to work on
a lawsuit for the firm of Abdullah Sheth.

The lawsuit was for a large sum (£40,000), and was
complicated to a high degree by disputes over bookkeeping details. Gandhi had to go through some severe study,
involving a self-given course in bookkeeping, before he
could understand it. Quite early in this operation he made
up his mind, and told his employer, that he would try to
settle it out of court if he could. This remained a fixed
principle in all his professional career, and most of his
cases were so settled. This was advisable because of the
great saving in fees, he thought, but also, and perhaps
chiefly, because the suit was between relatives who had
been and ought to be friends.

Some three days after he had landed in Durban, his
employer took him to a magistrate's court to see how it
worked. Gandhi in those days wore his English clothes,
but with an Indian turban—like the *pugree* of Bengal—
on his head. Those who wear the turban never take it off
indoors or out; decorum requires that it be kept on, as is
the case nowadays with the Gandhi cap. The English
custom of removing the hat on entering a house or courtroom is thus directly at variance with Indian proprieties.
Gandhi entered the court with his turban on and kept it
on, though he noticed the magistrate staring at him.
Eventually the magistrate asked him to remove the turban; he refused and left the courtroom.

There was quite a little row about this incident; Gandhi wrote to the papers defending his right to wear an
Indian turban at all times, and a controversy arose which
made him known in Natal sooner than he might have
been otherwise. In this dilemma his self-respect as an

Indian was, he felt, at stake, but he was willing to compromise by wearing an English hat—which, of course, he would have removed indoors in the English manner. His employer was very much against that, and Gandhi took his advice, wearing his turban thereafter as a sort of badge of independence. ("If you wear a hat you will look like a waiter," his employer had said.)

When he felt that he understood the lawsuit well enough, Gandhi notified Abdullah Sheth that he was ready to go to Pretoria, the capital of the Transvaal, where the case was to be tried. Abdullah was anxious; the Transvaal was even more difficult than Natal for Indians; the journey was long; there was the question of where Gandhi could stay in Pretoria. The young barrister made light of the difficulties and set forth in the train with a first-class ticket.

When the train reached Maritzburg, the capital of Natal, a white passenger came along, saw him in the first-class compartment, went away, and came back again with some railroad officials. Gandhi was ordered to go into the "van compartment," where Indians usually traveled. He refused. A constable was summoned, and he was forcibly removed from the first-class compartment. Because he refused on principle to travel in any other manner, he had to sit in the railway station at Maritzburg all night long in the bitter cold. In the morning he sent telegrams to the railway management and to Abdullah Sheth in Durban, who took appropriate steps; the Indian merchants of Maritzburg, informed by telegram, came to see him to tell him their own troubles of the same order; when the next evening's train arrived a sleeping-berth had been reserved for him, and he accepted it. If he had been willing to pay for bedding and a berth in the first place, the incident would not have occurred, but he had been eager to avoid undue expense to his employers.

In the sleeping-berth Gandhi arrived the next morning at Charlestown, the end of the railway, where he had to take a stagecoach to Johannesburg. Here were more difficulties. At first the coach agent wanted to refuse him a passage, but on Gandhi's insistence allowed him to come along—not inside the coach with the other passengers, but on the box outside, along with the coachman. The young barrister "pocketed the insult," as he said, but later on in the day when the coach agent wanted to come out for air and told Gandhi to sit on the footboard so that he (the agent) could sit by the coachman and smoke, Gandhi refused. The man thereupon proceeded to beat him up—a thorough assault, witnessed by the passengers, who protested in vain. At the night stop (Standerton), Gandhi was met by Indian merchants who kept him overnight, and in the morning he was given a seat, without incident, on a new coach with a new conductor.

At Johannesburg there was a fresh incident: he could not be admitted to the Grand National Hotel. When he found his Indian merchant friends at last (having missed them at the station), they explained to him that no Indian could stay in any hotel in this country. They warned him that the Dutch Transvaal was much worse than English Natal, and that on his journey to Pretoria on the following day he would be obliged to travel third-class: it was an iron rule.

Gandhi was as obstinate then, in his gentle way, as he was ever afterwards. It was a matter of principle, and he would not give in. He wrote to the station-master of

Johannesburg and stated his intention, then proceeded to buy a first-class ticket. The station-master, a Dutchman from Holland, sold the ticket, but asked Gandhi not to involve him in any trouble that might result.

It was a lucky day, apparently, in that two fair-minded Europeans stood by the brave little challenger. When the guard on the train, taking tickets, ordered Gandhi to leave the first class, the only fellow passenger in the compartment happened to be an Englishman who defended Gandhi and would not allow him to be evicted. The guard said: "Well, if you want to travel with a coolie—!" The train reached Pretoria without further incident.

In Pretoria there was nobody to meet the traveler. He stood in the dimly lighted station and wondered what to do, where to go. He waited until all the passengers had departed and then approached the ticket-collector with his problem. Was there any small hotel where he might find lodging for the night? The ticket-collector knew of none.

At this point another providential stranger befriended him. It was an American Negro who intervened and said he knew of a small hotel, owned by an American, where Gandhi would be accepted. The Negro took the traveler to Johnston's Family Hotel, where Mr. Johnston agreed to give him a room if he was willing to eat his dinner there rather than in the dining-room. Gandhi took the room; he was learning fast. Mr. Johnston consulted his European customers, found that they were quite willing to eat in the same room with Gandhi, and brought him downstairs with apologies.

On the next day Gandhi waited upon Abdullah Sheth's attorney, Mr. A. W. Baker, who found board and lodging for him in the house of a poor woman willing to put up with the ignominy of an Indian guest for thirty-five shillings a week.

We hear a good deal about Mr. A. W. Baker from Gandhi, not as a lawyer but because it seems to have been Baker's desire to convert him to Christianity. Baker was deeply religious and afterwards gave up his law practice to become a missionary; even before that he was a lay preacher. He had built a church in Pretoria at his own expense, and among other things he had a daily prayer-meeting, to which he invited Gandhi at once. Those who frequented the prayer-meeting included a number of ladies who befriended young Gandhi, and, among others, Mr. Michael Coates, a Quaker, who seems to have become one of Gandhi's best friends in those early years.

But Christianity was not really for Gandhi, then or afterwards, because its central theological doctrine was unsympathetic to him, and indeed beyond his capacity to believe—as it would be for most Hindus. Brought up to think that all men are sons of God, how could Gandhi at twenty-four suddenly concentrate the whole world-wide divinity of Hinduism into one historic figure? The exclusive divinity of Jesus of Nazareth was the first difficulty, but another, not far behind it, was the attribution of the soul to human beings alone. Gandhi's instinctive belief was in the unity of all life, which included animals as well, and although he was not at that time very conversant with the doctrines of Hinduism, he must have had an awareness from childhood (as all Hindus have) of the deeply rooted convictions concerned with metempsychosis, the cycle of death and rebirth. Whether he fully knew or believed in his own religion or not, too much of it was implanted in his consciousness for him to abandon it for another so different. And indeed, the principal result of some months of association with these devout Christians, who gave him books to read and prayed for his conversion, was to turn him back upon his own religion with a renewed interest in it.

If, as I believe, the genius of Gandhi was primarily religious, those early days in Pretoria must have been among the formative experiences of his life. He was face to face, for the first time, with a proselytizing effort—nobody in England had tried to convert him to anything—and a steady running argument that sharpened his perceptions while arousing his deeper religious instinct, his Vaishnava heritage. He was informed of all the Christian doctrines about sin and redemption, the vicarious redemption through Jesus, which seemed to him—who wished to be redeemed "not from the consequences of sin but from sin itself"—inapplicable to reality. He even encountered one zealous missioner, a member of the Plymouth Brethren, who permitted himself a certain latitude in transgression on the ground that Jesus had already atoned for it for him. The books Gandhi was given to read were full of doctrine, none of which moved him at all. The Sermon on the Mount came to be a very important part of his consciousness in the years ahead, but neither in the early days nor later could he accept the Christian theology.

Gandhi, so earnest and hard-working, had never until this time found himself able to study religious literature or think what it was that he did believe. He had always been busy with his duties. Now he had little to do, other lawyers were working on the Abdullah-Tyeb law-suit, and his services were not, for the moment, required. Thus he found, originally through Christian influences, but afterwards through Mohammedanism and Hinduism, a whole world of thought congenial to him and opening up vistas toward what was to be, at last, his own religion, his own kind of universalist Hinduism.

His experiences on the way to Pretoria had given him a fairly good idea of the status of Indians in the Transvaal, and he wished, during this period of waiting for work, to do what he could about it. He went to Tyeb Sheth, the person against whom his lawsuit was intended, and made friends, a characteristic move on his part. With his help Gandhi called a meeting of all the Indians in the Transvaal capital. It was held in the house of a leading Moslem merchant, and Gandhi made a speech—the first he had ever made.

That, too, was characteristic: he wanted to help the Indians, but he began by telling them what they themselves should do. His most earnest plea was made for truthfulness in business. He had learned with dismay that many of the Indian merchants regarded truth as having little place in business, and his effort was to convince them not only that truth was essential, in business as elsewhere, but that any lapse from it would do the Indians as a community much harm—that a single merchant in a strange land might harm all his fellow Indians by untruthfulness. He went on (of course) to hygiene and sanitation, urging them to reform in these respects. He asked them to obliterate all the distinctions of religion and race brought over from India (Hindu, Moslem, Parsee, Christian, Punjabi, Madrassi, and the like). He suggested the formation of an association on a permanent basis to defend the rights of the Indians and to put their case before the authorities from time to time.

It was a sort of model Gandhi speech—he was to make countless others of the same kind before the end. It concluded, of course, with his offer to do anything he could.

The interest aroused was considerable; the association was formed; three young men went to Gandhi and asked him for lessons in English. Gandhi, who had been studying the railway regulations of the Transvaal, wrote in the association's name to the railway authorities and told them that even under their own rules the Indians were entitled to travel in any class for which they bought a ticket. The authorities replied that first and second class would henceforth be open to Indians who were "properly dressed"—a matter of interpretation for the ticket-seller.

Thus began, on the smallest scale, and unnoticed by any but a handful of Indians in Pretoria, the mission of Mahatma Gandhi. It was what he was soon to call "public work," a kind of service for which he would never accept any emolument. He had never done it before, and it is doubtful if he had any idea of what it was to lead him into as the years rolled by. And yet the germ of almost all his "public work" is in that one meeting and one speech in 1893. The Indians were to discipline themselves, tell the truth, be clean and keep their quarters clean, learn English, forget their internal differences—all this so as to achieve self-respect and set themselves free. So far as externals go, this was pretty much what Gandhi asked of them for the next fifty-odd years. He did not think of this as political, and indeed it would be difficult to find any political overtones or implications in what he had to say. It was rather an effort for the general welfare of the Indians, beginning (as was Gandhi's way) with the Indians themselves.

There were, as he was learning every day and every week, endless disabilities, humiliations, and hardships for the Indians of the Transvaal and the Orange Free State. Indians were actually excluded from the Free State, except in designated menial jobs; in the Transvaal they suffered under crippling legislation. They had no vote and could not own land except in special "locations," as they were called, and Gandhi said that in practice even the locations were not theirs. They had to pay a three-pound poll tax even to enter the Transvaal. They could not go out at night after nine o'clock without a special permit, and they could not walk on the public footpaths, but must take to the road with the beasts. On one occasion Gandhi was assaulted by a policeman somewhere near President Kruger's house for walking on the footpath—something he had done often before without incident. These rules were administered according to the whims of the police, and as the Indians had in effect no means of redress, treatment of them wavered between indulgence and brutality.

Gandhi's growing concern over the predicament of the Indians was checked for a while by practical reasons: he now had to deal with the lawsuit between Abdullah Sheth and his cousin Tyeb Sheth. Gandhi was employed in the preparation of Abdullah's case for the attorney, who accepted some things and rejected others. The attorney then briefed the counsel, who also accepted some parts of the presentation and rejected others. Gandhi says that this practical work was for him an education in the law, as well as in bookkeeping, translation, and other tasks.

He was, however, set upon an amiable solution of the problem as he saw the fees mounting and the expenses accumulating. Patiently and well he worked on Tyeb Sheth, the friendly enemy, and upon the various counsel, until he was able to get their consent to the appointment of an arbitrator; the case was argued, and Gandhi's client won. It was then his self-appointed task to persuade Abdullah, his employer, to allow payment of the claim in installments, and to persuade the proud Tyeb Sheth to agree. He says that if the whole sum had been exacted at once, Tyeb would have been bankrupt. He had his way: the installment system over a long period of years was adopted, and the peaceful outcome was in the end a solace to both sides, strongly as they had resisted it. It was Gandhi's habit thereafter, in all his cases, to try for such peaceful settlements—a strange form of law practice, but one that suited his peculiar talent.

Gandhi's year was up, and he prepared to go home after the case was settled. It had been a momentous year not only in his discoveries, but also in the arousing of his religious consciousness. He had read Tolstoy's *The Kingdom of God Is within You,* which penetrated his being as none of the arguments of orthodox Christianity had succeeded in doing. Tolstoy's argument (that governments, police, armies, and so on would be unnecessary if men would live by the Sermon on the Mount) was in harmony with Gandhi's natural feeling, and though he had not yet formulated an ideal, there cannot be much doubt that Tolstoy gave him a mighty push along the way toward it. It was not until 1909 that Gandhi dared to write to Tolstoy, but the influence began, according to his own account, in that first year in South Africa. The brilliance and bitterness of Tolstoy's attack upon Church and State, his slashing, scornful descriptions of the difference between word and deed among Christians, must burn deep into anybody who reads the book, and the power of the writer is such that objections do not arise until afterwards. Common sense will be stubborn enough to inquire, a day or so after one has finished the book, how in this world we know it can be possible to keep public order without any form of police. Tolstoy's answer—that if all obeyed the teachings of Christ all would be well—is no doubt quite true, but does not apply to any existing situation in human society. My belief is that Gandhi himself, in the course of his long pilgrimage, learned a great deal about the obstinacy of facts, and that his early burning enthusiasm for the Tolstoy doctrine was somewhat modified. He said to me, two days before he died: "Mind you, no ordinary government can get along without the use of force."

For the youth in South Africa, however, the blessings of experience (if blessings they be) were yet to come. He took from Tolstoy, with the utmost eagerness, the idea that a literal obedience to precept (the Sermon on the Mount, the *Gita*) would extricate him from the worst of the human predicament. The time was not far off when he would set himself to this literal obedience to precept, this adherence to the texts, as if to a map and a compass.

2

Gandhi went back to Durban and made his arrangements to go home. Abdullah Sheth arranged an all-day farewell for him, with a good many of the Indians of Durban present. In the course of the farewell party Gandhi became aware—by a chance paragraph in a newspaper that fell under his eye—of the "Indian Franchise Bill" of the Natal legislature. It was a bill withdrawing the right to vote from Indians, and had apparently already almost passed. Gandhi, in amazement, asked if his Indian friends of Durban had done nothing about it. They had not. They were more or less reconciled to their status; they felt that it was no use to struggle; they had paid little attention to the matter. He tried to tell them the importance of the franchise and the seriousness of their situation if they lost it. Their answer was a touching clamor for him to stay with them and tell them what to do.

Gandhi accepted for one month, on condition that they find the funds for a struggle against the Franchise Bill. He himself would accept no payment for public work, but the costs of printing, research, law consultations, and travel must be paid; moreover, one man could not do all the work; there must be volunteers.

As always when he called for volunteers, he got them. Having agreed to delay his departure for one month (which was to last for years), he flung himself into the work. He had discovered that the young Indians born in South Africa were for the most part Christians and did not associate much with the Moslem and Hindu Indians from India. He resolved to claim them for his work because they were young and to some degree educated; he actually succeeded in getting a good number of them to volunteer.

The first step was a telegraphed request to the Speaker of the Legislature to delay further debate on the Franchise Bill until the Indians could be heard. Then there was the drafting and copying out of the petition itself, with three handwritten copies for the legislature and an extra one for the press. The Speaker had given them only two days, and Gandhi with his volunteers worked night as well as day. When the two days were up, the Indian petition was presented in the legislature, read, and discussed; it appeared in the press; it created a stir; but the Franchise Bill was passed.

Such a last-minute failure was of the Gandhian variety: it only encouraged those involved to further effort. The Indians of Durban, divided into dozens of small, conflicting groups, had come together as one group for the first time, and this result was worth the failure. They now decided on a petition to London, to the Secretary of State for the Colonies (Lord Ripon), which would be signed by as many as possible of the Indians of Natal.

This was a much bigger undertaking, for Natal was huge and the villages were widely scattered. Gandhi's volunteers had a task equal to their utmost capacity. Aside from the central facts of Indian unity, organization, and communal effort, all of which were new in South Africa, the brief campaign brought out a number of novelties full of promise for the future. For example, the young men born in South Africa, many or most of whom had become Christians, once alienated from the other Indians, had come out for Gandhi, worked for him, and followed him. This may initially have been (and probably was) because of his London English, his London clothes, the fact that he was a barrister and a credit to the community; but his powers of gentle, persistent persuasion must have come into play already. Ten thousand signatures were obtained to the petition in two weeks. One thousand copies of it were printed for distribution in India, England, and elsewhere; the press was kept fully informed; both the *Times* in London and the *Times of India* (Bombay) supported the Indian claim to the vote. So far as England and India were concerned, this was their first real acquaintance with the questions arising out of racial prejudice in South Africa.

After the excitement of the month past it proved impossible for Gandhi to leave Natal. Too many people and things depended upon him. The Indians of Durban would not let him go. As he would not accept payment for "public work," the merchants banded together and guaranteed him enough professional work as a lawyer to stay another year. It was his desire, for quite impersonal reasons, to live in a manner befitting a London barrister, to travel first-class, and to compel respect; to do this he needed about three hundred pounds a year, and the sum was provided.

He went through a series of difficulties before he could be admitted as an advocate of the Supreme Court of Natal. The Law Society, made up entirely of Europeans, opposed his admission to the end. The Chief Justice made short shrift of their objections, declared that the law did not distinguish between colored and white people, and admitted Gandhi to take the oath at once. As soon as he had done so, the Chief Justice said: "You must now take off your turban, Mr. Gandhi." And this time Gandhi yielded. His turban, which had become a kind of symbol of his resistance to the oppression of Indians, did not seem to him important enough in this juncture to risk the loss of his place at the court.

He proceeded at once to the formation of a permanent organization among the Indians and, after some discussion, decided to call it the Natal Indian Congress. The choice of a name was delicate business; the Indian National Congress, at home in India, had already begun to irk conservative and imperialist opinion, though its activity was innocuous enough; and yet Gandhi felt that no other name could give the flavor of an all-embracing organization from which no Indian should be barred. Such nationalism as existed in India was already firmly associated with the word "Congress." Therefore, although he realized that he was running counter to much conservative and even moderate opinion, Gandhi adopted the controversial name.

The enthusiasm at the beginning was great, and there was no difficulty in obtaining the necessary subscriptions and donations from members. But those who had signed for contributions were not always prompt in paying them, and a good part of the work of Gandhi and his volunteers had to be wasted on collection of sums due. This, however, he insisted upon; one of his lifelong principles was to pay cash and never incur debts for any form of "public work." This principle was accompanied by another: he never wished to have more money in hand than was necessary. Between these two firm pillars—no debts and no surplus—he so built the Natal Indian Congress that it was steadily solvent for at least twenty years. Receipts were given for every sum, however small; accounts were kept with the greatest care. "Without properly kept accounts," Gandhi said, "it is impossible to maintain truth in its pristine purity."

Meetings of the Congress were held regularly, sometimes once a week and never less than once a month. Gandhi taught the members the rules of procedure—all new to them, of course; he was the only one who knew these things—and they learned eagerly. A library, a debating society, a special subsidiary body to bring together the educated young men born in South Africa—all these were quickly brought into being. The effort to state the case for the Indians naturally fell principally upon Gandhi, and he produced at this time two pamphlets for the Congress: *An Appeal to Every Briton in South Africa* and *The Indian Franchise—An Appeal*. Both went out far and wide, not only in South Africa, but to England and India, and evoked many expressions of sympathy. The question was ceasing to be local and becoming what it really was in fact, both general and fundamental.

At this stage of development the inevitable happened: Gandhi came into contact with the larger mass of Indians in South Africa, the indentured laborers. He had been aware of them all the time, but the nature of his occupations had kept him from any acquaintance with them. His work had thrown him entirely with the prosperous merchants and their staffs, but what he had already done was known throughout the Indian population.

One day a Tamil workman, trembling and weeping, appeared in his office. His mouth was bleeding and two front teeth had been knocked out. He held his turban in his hand deferentially—Mr. Gandhi was a barrister!— and poured forth his story. Gandhi, of course, did not understand Tamil, but his clerk was from southern India and translated for him. The man had been severely beaten by his master, a well-known European. Gandhi sent him to a doctor for a certificate of the injuries, and then took him to a magistrate, who issued a summons for the offending master.

The law governing indentured laborers was severe: a man could not leave his employment without risking criminal proceedings and imprisonment. It was, in fact, a form of slavery, mitigated by many circumstances (in-

cluding the time limit), but akin to slavery in that the
man had no freedom of action. Gandhi, who knew the
law, did not wish to see the brutal European master punished; he only wanted the victim released from that particular indenture and transferred, if possible, to another.
He secured the agreement of the European master (who
by that time was probably rather frightened) and then
went to the Protector of Indentured Laborers, a public
official, who released the man to another indenture. Gandhi, out of his slender acquaintance among Europeans,
found a new master willing to take the man.

The victim in the case was called Balasundaram, a
name Gandhi never forgot. The poor man, physically suffering and mentally in despair, had run to Gandhi's office because it was the only place he had ever heard of
where a poor coolie from southern India might be given
justice or protection. It was chance, perhaps, but chance
pregnant with consequences. Balasundaram played a brief
but decisive part in history because he acted, all unwit-
tingly, as the key to Gandhi's greater mission.

The episode was repeated and magnified; it became
legend overnight; there was a man, actually an Indian
sahib, a barrister, a man of the great, who did not dis-
dain to care for and to defend a poor beaten coolie. The
story went rapidly to southern India, to Madras itself,
and succeeding waves of Indian immigration were told,
even before they left India, that Gandhi was their friend.
As for Natal itself, the indentured laborers adopted him
at once, and streamed through his office from then onward. Gandhi's immense popularity in southern India,
which actually preceded his full recognition in the north,
came originally from the great legend (or great truth)
exemplified in the story of Balasundaram.

He was himself very deeply moved. Not only the suffering of the laborer, but the humility of the man—the fact that he held his headgear in his hand—struck deep into Gandhi's heart. He felt, as he had felt before, that those who had no help elsewhere were the people he most desired to help. The pathos of the headgear struck him more particularly because he had gone through such a series of incidents concerned with his own. The humiliation to which he had objected was here accepted as natural by the stricken man, the defenseless. Gandhi had asked him at once to resume his scarf, and Balasundaram had done so hesitantly, but with a glow of pleasure. Such small things were Gandhi's secret power, more than his external skills in law or action. There was no indentured laborer in Natal who did not know all about this within a few days.

3

As he conducted the campaign of the Natal Indian Congress and simultaneously earned his living at the bar, Gandhi continued to pursue the religious interests that had been aroused by the Christians of Pretoria. He continued to associate with Christian missionary friends, though in Durban the chief of them (Mr. Spencer Walton, head of the South African General Mission, and his wife) made no attempt to convert him. Christian books were available to him in numbers, but he also began now to study his own religion more carefully than ever before. His great friend Raychandra, in Bombay (whom he always called Raychandbhai—"Brother Raychand"), was of great use and considerable influence by correspondence during this period (1893–6) and afterwards. Gandhi had met Raychand on his return from London and had

been subjugated by the wit, learning, and character of
the man, only two or three years older than himself, who
could simultaneously conduct a jewelry firm and write
poetry, study Hindu Scriptures and read modern European literature. Raychand had the faculty, which must
have been fairly common among the Brahmins of ancient times, the possessor of which is called a *Shatava-
dhani*—that is, he could remember word for word, syllable by syllable, whatever was said to him and could
repeat it back, no matter in what order or in what language. It was by this method, of course, that the Brahmins preserved the Hindu Scriptures through the many
long centuries before the invention of writing—by complicated technical feats of acrostic, inverted order, and
the like, guaranteeing that the sacred words (which were
a Brahmin secret and the basis of Brahmin dominion)
would never be lost from memory. Gandhi's fascination
with Raychandra's extraordinary personality had been
keen in their actual meetings in Bombay; it became a
strong devotion, almost a pupil-teacher devotion, during
the years in South Africa when Raychand counseled him
by letter.

Under that counsel he read some of the Hindu Scriptures (in English, of course), particularly the *Upanishads* in a translation put out by the Theosophical Society. He read Max Müller and some other writers on
India; there were some vernacular books in Gujarati on
religious subjects. His regard for his own religion and his
desire to know more of it were growing. At the same
time he read more books on Islamic subjects, Washington Irving's *Life of Mahomet* being one. And those pamphlets or polemical works which Tolstoy had been pour-
ing out—*The Gospel in Brief* and *What to Do?* were

two of them; *What Is Art?* came a year later—were almost as important as any Scripture to Gandhi. Oddly enough he never discovered, throughout his life, how much Tolstoy was a literary phenomenon—how little Tolstoy really signified in the action of life, the enactment of precept, the doing of the thing thought. Gandhi was simple-minded. If a man said that the Sermon on the Mount was the one single rule, he believed that to this man it was the one single rule. He endeavored thereafter, in increasing degree, to make it so for himself. He never found out that the man who made the preachment could not himself obey it. He seems always to have assumed the total sincerity of others as he extended the areas of literal sincerity in himself. Thus he came in the end to the essential error of all great souls: "I am a creature of nothing, devoid of special faculties for achievement, and yet I can do it, therefore why can all others not do it? What I, poor limited creature, can do—in disciplinary resolutions, that is—must be much easier for others, or at least as easy." This was his greatest fallacy, and the measure of his failure in South Africa, India, and the world. He thought all others could do what he did, because in fact he thought all others were superior to him in capacity to do things. This error was fatal: it puts him with Socrates, the Lord Gautama Buddha, and the Lord Jesus of Nazareth, the three most spectacular failures known in human history. All of them believed that other men could do what they did. They were wrong, and so was Gandhi.

He had now completed three years in South Africa, and it was quite apparent that he would have to stay a long time if he hoped to bring to any good result the work that he had initiated. He made a compact with his

Moslem friends in Durban: they would permit him to go home to India to collect his family and his possessions, such as they were, and to come back on the same terms as before. He picked two devoted volunteers to run the Natal Indian Congress during his absence and set sail for Bombay.

CHAPTER THREE

SATYAGRAHA

ON the way to India, Gandhi quite characteristically studied two Indian languages, Tamil and Urdu, which he felt he ought to know, and both of them from or with British officers of the ship. At all stages of his life British people instinctively liked him, tried to make friends with him, helped him in all his efforts. He reciprocated the feeling, and it may truthfully be said that the British never had in all their wondrous history a more loyal and loving rebel than Gandhi. He did not learn Tamil, but he got to the point where he could read it quite easily; Urdu came with less difficulty, but he never got it right either, in spite of some years in jail afterwards when he had ample opportunity for study.

In India he did his best—aside from his domestic arrangements about moving the family to South Africa—to make known to all the questions that now interested him.

He began by writing a pamphlet on the Indians in South Africa; it had a green cover and was thereafter known as the Green Pamphlet. Copies went to every newspaper in India and England, to every person of importance in the Indian National Congress, to officials, and to persons assumed to be interested. It made a great stir and was commented upon editorially by the newspapers in both countries. Reuters sent a summary to London, and their London office sent an even briefer summary to Natal—for which Gandhi was to pay by much peril and anguish.

He sent out these pamphlets (one thousand of them) by means of volunteers in his own native place, Rajkot, but in this case he made use of small children. It was the first time he had thought of asking children to do this kind of work. Later on he was to rely upon them repeatedly for such enterprises; they were eager, happy to do it, and felt themselves made important by trying.

At this moment there was an outbreak of plague in Bombay, and Gandhi volunteered his services, as usual, thus making his first acquaintance with latrines and sanitary arrangements in Indian houses. He found, on his inspection tours, that the houses of the well-to-do were less sanitary than those of the very poor, and in particular of the untouchables, whom he saw now for the first time in their own homes. Gandhi's descriptions of the latrines and urinals of some upper-class houses are to be read now with amazement: it does not seem possible that Hindus of the highest caste could live, eat, and sleep in such a perpetual stench, and yet he saw and smelled for himself.

He also met friends who would be useful thereafter, especially in Bombay—Sir Pherozeshah Mehta, the great Bombay lawyer, and other Parsees and Hindus of note. The principal one, the one who had most influence upon him, was Gokhale, the head of the Indian National Congress, who welcomed him as a son. Gokhale was by all accounts a very remarkable man, and without his spadework, his fundamental organization of the Indian consciousness, it is possible that Gandhi could not have fulfilled his own mission. In any case the instinctive communication of the two men, wide apart in age, was immediate, and Gandhi ever afterwards referred to Gokhale

as his "political guru," his master in all those matters
which had to do with public work.

There was a visit to Madras: wild enthusiasm. The
story of Balasundaram had been spread throughout the
Tamil and Telugu country. Gandhi was the protector of
the slave laborers of South Africa, most of whom had
come from the province of Madras. He could not speak
to these people in their own language, but was obliged to
use English, as he did for many decades thereafter in
southern India. But, said he, "What barrier is there that
love cannot break?"

In Bengal it was different: Gandhi had to wait for
hours to see important editors or persons who could help
the Indians of South Africa. The fact was that scarcely
any Bengalis—perhaps not even one—had gone to South
Africa, so that the question seemed very remote from the
offices in Calcutta. As usual, Gandhi found an Englishman (Mr. Saunders, editor of *The Englishman*) who
espoused his cause, gave him office room and space in the
newspaper and everything he required for the presentation of his case. But then his six months' leave came to
an end, and cablegrams from Durban urged him to return. He left Calcutta for Bombay, collected his wife,
two sons, and a nephew, and set sail in December 1896
to return to South Africa.

2

Gandhi tells us how he dressed his wife and children
on this journey. He wanted to compel the Europeans to
respect Indians as Indians. Even at that time he cared
little or nothing about himself, but he regarded himself
as representative of the community, almost a symbol of

the struggle (as indeed he was), and therefore he wanted
to represent. His wife and children could not really dress
as Europeans, but they could dress as Parsees, which was
the nearest thing in India to European. This meant coat,
trousers, and shoes for the boys, a Parsee sari and shoes
and stockings for poor Kasturbai. None of them had ever
worn shoes before, and it was a great pain: their toes got
sore and the stockings smelled of perspiration, offensive to
them. Gandhi also made them use the knife and the fork,
which always do seem (even today) an abomination to
Indians who wish to eat with clean hands.

The boat belonged to Abdullah Sheth's firm and made
straight from Bombay to Durban, taking only eighteen
days instead of the six weeks of the preceding voyage. At
Durban it was delayed for quarantine: there had been
cholera in Bombay. This was comprehensible, of course,
but during the five extra days ordered by the doctors
(eighteen of the voyage, five in quarantine) quite different themes began to be heard. It was not merely that
twenty-three days were required for cholera to develop.
It seemed that Mr. Gandhi was the point at issue.

The Natal white people (and I cannot make out from
the evidence what the Government of Natal was doing,
if it was doing anything) had made up their minds that
Gandhi was a trouble-maker and should not be permitted to land. They wanted him and all the persons on his
ship and on another ship that anchored at the same time,
also full of Indians, to return to India at once. During
the five days of quarantine, some agents of the white as-
sociations went among the passengers of the two ships
saying: if you return to India you may possibly get your
passage money back, but if you insist on staying here you
will be shoved into the sea. Gandhi counteracted this as

best he could by moving among the passengers and telling them to be calm and wait.

An ultimatum was served on the passengers at Christmas: they would return to India or run the risk of death. All, without exception, said that they stuck to their right to land at Port Natal—a matter of principle in which Gandhi had had ample time to instruct them.

Gandhi was the cause of the trouble, as became amply evident when they landed. When there was no further legal excuse for keeping the ships outside, they were authorized to enter the harbor and disembark their passengers. Gandhi, however, was a very special case. A message came aboard from the English lawyer for the Abdullah firm, saying that Gandhi and his wife and children should not attempt to get off the boat until it got dark, as feeling was excited against him. He agreed to this.

Then another of the Abdullah lawyers, a man named Laughton, came to Gandhi and said that it would be best for Mrs. Gandhi and the children to disembark, take a carriage, and go straight to the house of the Indian friend (Rustomji) with whom they were supposed to lodge. Gandhi himself should take his chances on foot. Gandhi agreed to this too.

Finally he was allowed to get off the boat. His wife and children had driven without incident to Rustomji's house. Gandhi got off with Mr. Laughton and walked a few feet, upon which some rowdy youths started shouting: "Gandhi! Gandhi!" and a crowd quickly assembled. Mr. Laughton summoned a rickshaw (a form of conveyance of which Gandhi thoroughly disapproved), but the rickshaw boy was frightened off by abuse and took to his heels. Gandhi and Mr. Laughton went on

walking. They were beset by the crowd and separated
(this was in broad daylight), and Gandhi was showered
with stones, brickbats, and rotten eggs. His turban was
torn off and he was severely beaten and kicked by the
mob. Then, as was always his case, an English person
saved him—in this case Mrs. Alexander, the wife of the
Superintendent of Police. She knew Gandhi, and, seeing
a little man beaten against an iron railing where he was
clinging, half-conscious, while the hoodlums assailed
him, she calmly stood beside him and opened up her
umbrella between the mob and Gandhi and herself.
The umbrella was strictly symbolic, but everybody in
the mob knew Mrs. Alexander and nobody dared attack
her. Gandhi was safe.

Alexander, the Police Superintendent, arrived in time
and got Gandhi off to Rustomji's house under guard,
but there again a mob formed with the plain intention of
lynching him. This time Alexander got him out of the
house by the back way, disguised as a police constable,
and meanwhile held the mob in leash by singing to them:

> *Hang old Gandhi*
> *On the sour apple tree.*

For two or three days thereafter Gandhi was kept in
the police station under guard, but when the storm blew
over, it was found that in reality it had benefited him.
None of the accusations against him was true. The white
people thought he had brought over all the Indians on
both the ships in the harbor: he had had nothing to do
with their migration, and in any case most of them were
old residents of Africa who had been to India on a visit.
The whites also blamed Gandhi for a very brief and mis-
leading article, sent by Reuters from India to England

and thence to South Africa, which gave a distorted version of what he had said of conditions in Natal. When
all this was cleared up, a sense of justice prevailed and
Gandhi was more esteemed than ever among the Natal
whites. He himself believed that his subsequent work
was aided, rather than hindered, by the episode.

3

He was at a very curious transition just at the end of
the nineteenth century. He was physically very lustful
(two of his sons were born in South Africa, and one he
delivered himself because the doctor was late). Yet he
had begun to think and feel that he could not fulfill his
appointed tasks unless he abstained totally from sexual
intercourse. This idea, very deep in Hinduism, is embodied in the word *brahmacharya*, "the learning of God,"
by which is meant self-control and an abnegation of sen-
sual appetite. *Brahmacharya* is recommended to all Hindus at the beginning and at the end of their lives (the
first and last of the four ages of man). Gandhi knew little of Hinduism, but this idea began to haunt him.

Furthermore, his ideas of his public duty were in a
state that cannot be called confused, but must be regarded
as evolving slowly. His loyalty to the British Raj was intense ("God save the Queen!") and remained so until
the great rebellious days of the 1920's. When the Boer
War came—it was inevitable and had been in preparation for years—Gandhi felt a general sympathy for the
Boers, but an overruling loyalty to England. It was
hardly even a conflict for him—he did not think that his
instinctive sympathy for the Boers made any difference:
the important thing was his born, sworn, and felt loyalty
to England. Thus he organized and led an Indian medi-

cal corps (over one thousand men), which served with
distinction, even under fire on some occasions (as at Spion
Kop), and received the thanks of the highest authorities.
The episode served to strengthen the prestige and therefore the bargaining position of the Indians in South Africa, but, as usual, this result was incidental to Gandhi's
original desire to give loyal service.

Medical service was, as a matter of fact, congenial to
Gandhi and remained one of his preoccupations. He had
started by nursing his own children, medically speaking,
and by actually delivering one of them. Then he found
himself able to give two hours a day to a free hospital in
which many poor Indians were treated. His lifelong interest in nursing thus arose naturally and gradually, so
that when the war came he was psychologically ready
for what he had to do. He always gave first importance
to these tasks, and in later days was quite capable of
keeping a whole cabinet or a whole empire waiting while
he took care of a poor leper. In fact, some of his "miracles" (like all legend-creators or legend-centers, Gandhi
had many miracles attributed to him) came from his simple nursing techniques. In the case of a little girl who had
been pronounced dead and whom he restored to life,
years later in India, he said with some asperity: "Miracle? Nonsense! I merely gave the child an enema." Giving enemas, applying bandages and poultices, caring for
the sick in every way imaginable, were parts of what he
felt to be his job. There is no doubt whatever that his
gentle voice, his great long tender hands, and his simple,
natural affection for all creatures had something to do
with the generally fortunate results of his nursing. He
could give comfort and peace even when he most lacked
it himself.

And he did lack it. *Brahmacharya* was by no means
easy for him. It took him years to achieve. He began to
try, by self-control and without formal vows, in 1901
after the Boer War was over. He did not feel strong
enough to take the final vow until 1906, which means
that for five years he repeatedly failed to overcome his
sexual desires. This battle, which so many great and good
men have engaged upon through the centuries, was perhaps harder for Gandhi than for anybody else we can
easily remember. St. Augustine was, by comparison, a
very poor second. (He prayed for chastity, but "Not
yet, Lord, not yet!" and was comfortably ensconced with
a mistress at the very time when his mother was arranging
his marriage.) Origen castrated himself. This Gandhi
would have abhorred as he abhorred every interference
with nature. But he did profoundly feel that the spirit
within him demanded a release from physical bondage,
that he must overcome the desires of the body, and that
only in such a release could his work be done. In this he
does not seem to have been influenced particularly by
Hindu Scriptures, though innumerable texts advocate
brahmacharya. It seems to have been by his own nature's
law—and he found the texts afterwards. At the very beginning of the struggle he told his poor, faithful Kasturbai, who had (by his own account) suffered so much
from the excesses of his lust, and she agreed that he
should make the attempt. Perhaps it was a relief to her.
At all events she must have been sure, as he declared so
often, that his sexual nature was entirely concentrated
upon her, and that he had never been unfaithful.

4

After the Boer War was over, Gandhi again returned to India. He wanted it to be a definitive return—he felt that he had been away long enough—but his friends of the Natal Indian Congress exacted from him a pledge that if they needed him again, he would come back to them. In the series of farewells given him, many expensive presents were bestowed upon him, all because he had worked for the community without pay. His conscience irked him over these gifts, some of which were extremely valuable, and he resolved to put them into a bank as a trust fund to support public work for the Indians in case of need. Kasturbai was very hard to persuade on this count, but as he had the children on his side he eventually won, and the objects of gold and diamonds were all put in trust. Later on he was grateful for the ease with which he could raise money on these gifts in cases of emergency.

In India his first interest was to attend the 1901 meeting of the Indian National Congress at Calcutta. This body, a curiosity in political history, was then sixteen years old. It had been founded by an Englishman, Allan Octavian Hume, who was its Secretary until 1907. Lord Dufferin, the Viceroy of the time, had actually wished to strengthen the Congress by making it more Indian, by asking Indians to preside over it and organize it. Its purposes were social and political: it was to canalize the rising nationalism of the Indians, both Hindu and Moslem, into ways of moderation and legality. It was to do what it could for the general welfare and to express, as much as possible, the wishes of the country. As illiteracy was then very widespread (well above the ninety per cent registered in later years), the inevitable result was that the Congress became an assembly of middle-class intellectuals, lawyers, merchants, and the like, who spoke for India in a notably timid and circumspect manner. Even so, it was the only national association that could speak for India at all, and Gandhi felt it to be the "life blood" of the country. The meeting of 1901 was his initiation: beyond a doubt he was incapable of realizing then what an instrument the Congress was to become in his own hands.

His main purpose was to present a resolution in support of the Indians of South Africa. But he had two or three days, first, to appreciate the physical difficulties of a vast meeting of his fellow countrymen. The lack of sanitation distressed him, and he would have cleaned the latrines himself if it had been possible; as it was, he contented himself with cleaning the one particular latrine that he was using. He did clerical work as a volunteer and kept his eyes and ears open. Much displeased him, and yet he felt a thrill of excitement at the thought of being present in a truly national assembly. When it came time to read his own resolution, it was late; all resolutions were passed unanimously anyhow; few persons listened to him or cared what was in the resolution; it went through without a dissenting vote because Gokhale, the great man of the Congress, had read and approved it.

After the Congress meeting Gandhi spent a month as Gokhale's guest. He was to remember this to the end. There were both good and bad in this month of Calcutta. Through Gokhale Gandhi met many eminent persons to whom he could preach his gospel of help for the Indians of South Africa, and he felt that this was abundantly useful. But on one occasion he went to the Temple of Kali, and was horrified at the blood sacrifice that took place there. The sheep or the lamb, he felt, was life even as the human being was life. He never reconciled himself to blood sacrifice and did his best to bring it to an end in India.

Finally, after a brief visit to Rangoon, he said his farewells to Gokhale and started for Bombay. For the first time, he wished to travel third-class in order to study the conditions of the Indian poor. Indian third-class then (and now) is incredibly dirty, overcrowded, and unsanitary. Gokhale did his best to dissuade Gandhi from this experiment, but without success. The little man had a tremendous obstinacy when he had made up his mind. He wanted to stop in four or five places, including Benares, and traveled by ordinary trains between them. Now, too, for the first time, he adopted ordinary Indian clothing, the shirt and *dhoti*, or wrapped skirt.

He recorded his shock at the conditions he found. From then on, whenever he was in India, with an interruption caused by his serious illness in 1918–19, he tried to travel third-class, partly as a protest against the conditions there and partly to inform himself of them. In later years the governmental authorities (both British and, later, Indian) went to great lengths to ensure cleanliness and decorum on any third-class carriage that Gandhi used. His ashes were eventually transported to the confluence of the sacred rivers in a special train made up entirely of third-class carriages.

In Benares, Gandhi was irritated, repelled, and in fact made downright angry by the dirt and money-grubbing he found around the temples, above all the Kashi Vishvanath (the Temple of the Master of the World). The dirty little lanes leading to the temple, the rubbishy little shops, the general atmosphere of paltry profiteering, disgusted him. He was to go to Benares afterwards, but only after he had become Mahatma and was revered by the multitude. Even then, years later, Benares repelled him.

He went to see Annie Besant, who had been ill and was only just convalescent. This brilliant and extraordinary creature had made her way through socialism and various other beliefs into theosophy, but in so doing had performed a genuine service to India by arousing the interest of young people in the literature and tradition of their own past. She used to make lecture tours all over India, and although as an Englishwoman she might have been supposed to belong to the colonial oppressor's bailiwick, she was in fact an important influence in the Indian renaissance, the revival of an awareness of India's glory. Gandhi had deep respect for her for these reasons, though he was not himself then or at any other time a member of the Theosophical Society.

Back in Bombay he tried to return to the bar, but it was not to be. The Indians of South Africa needed him and sent an urgent cablegram: Joseph Chamberlain was coming to South Africa; Gandhi must "return immediately." He had given his pledge on leaving Durban, and now he had no choice. This time he took with him four or five young men who wanted to go and might be useful in his work there. Among these was his second cousin Maganlal Gandhi, who was to prove one of the most useful lieutenants in the great struggle now about to begin.

Gandhi arrived in Durban just in time to draw up the paper and present it. Chamberlain had come to Africa to get a big monetary gift and to reconcile, if possible, the lately embattled British and Boers. He had short shrift for the Indians, declared that the government in London could not control the self-governing colonies, and advised the Indians to "placate" the Europeans if they wished to live in Africa at all.

From Natal it was necessary for Gandhi to go immediately to the Transvaal, where Chamberlain was due next, and do the same thing for the Transvaal Indian community. The Transvaal, smarting under defeat, was a far rougher and tougher country for an Indian than Natal. In the first place, Indians could not get a permit to enter the country without much exercise of influence and (in many cases) heavy bribery. The ravages of war had been severe, and the British conquerors had brought in a whole new set of officers from India, Ceylon, and elsewhere, who were new to the country and operated in an autocratic manner. Gandhi got his permit by asking his old friend Police Superintendent Alexander, who had once saved his life. But in Pretoria he found that the new Asiatic Office (manned by British officers from India) was adamant against him: he would not be permitted to see Chamberlain or take any part in the affair, and in fact his permit to enter the Transvaal was questioned. He drew up the petition and had it read to Chamberlain by another Indian barrister, a Christian.

But what he saw in the Transvaal in a few days made him feel that the Indians there needed him far more than did the Indians of Natal. He resolved to stay, to set up offices as a barrister in Johannesburg, and to give as much time as he could to the protection of the Indians. To his surprise the Law Society of the Transvaal made no objection (he was, of course, the only Indian) and the

Supreme Court admitted him quite tranquilly as an advocate.

His first task was to expose the shameless way in which the Indians were being fleeced for re-entry permits. Many had left the Transvaal during the war; to come back they were compelled to pay large sums, up to one hundred pounds each, for the permit. Gandhi patiently collected the evidence and then took it to the Police Commissioner. A trial ensued in which the guilty officers were acquitted by a jury, but after such a thorough exposure that the abuses came to an end and the officers themselves were dismissed from their employ. In this respect the Indians enjoyed relief and Gandhi's prestige as their protector, already great, rose to new levels.

Gradually Gandhi's system of living began to be patriarchal, even though he was in fact only in his early thirties. He took his office clerks to live with him, along with the young men he had brought from India and also, from time to time, various Englishmen and other Europeans whom he wished to know better. He was simplifying his existence in every way possible, materially speaking, and these visitors or guests had to conform to the rules of the house. He was up every morning at six (which he seemed to regard as a sinfully late hour), and he had learned from some book to skip breakfast as being unnecessary; he was now becoming not only a vegetarian, but a strict dietician with a liking for experiment. It was just at this time, in Johannesburg, that he embarked on the diet of fruit and nuts which sustained him for a good many years thereafter. His religious interests were deepening, and he never ceased to read books on Hinduism at this time.

Among his helpers two European girls were pre-eminent. The first was Miss Dick, a Scottish girl who had just come to South Africa and who declared herself quite willing to work for an Indian. Gandhi found her invaluable, and was happy to give her away in marriage when she became Mrs. MacDonald. Next came Miss Schlesin, a South African girl of German origin, afterwards a teacher in the public schools. She was frank, impetuous, and sincere, and at a time when Ghandi and almost all his co-workers were in jail she ran the whole Indian movement herself, practically singlehanded. Gandhi esteemed her work more highly than that of almost any other of his followers. She refused to accept more than ten pounds a month and grew angry when he tried to raise her pay. She came to him at the age of seventeen and stayed throughout the days of turmoil.

The next step was the foundation of a weekly journal, *Indian Opinion*, started in 1904, in which for the next ten years Gandhi poured out his thought and feeling on all the subjects of interest to the Indian community. He was neither the proprietor nor the editor, but a great part of his earnings as a barrister went into the support of the paper, and it was known throughout South Africa that he wrote the editorials. He was himself convinced that his success in South Africa—and *satyagraha* itself, voluntary sacrifice—became possible only through the existence of this newspaper. He received an enormous mail from all parts of the country as a result of what he wrote, and that his words were so widely read was to prove vital in the subsequent development. At first the paper came out in English, Gujarati, Tamil, and Hindi, but Gandhi soon became aware that only the first two of these were really read, and the editions were then, at his insistence, reduced to English and Gujarati, both of which were native languages to him. *Indian Opinion* was his primary instrument in the struggle for the next ten years.

His immediate task in "public work" was the defense of the poor Indians, most of them indentured laborers who had served out their time, against dispossession of their land. The "coolie location," outside Johannesburg, was dirty and neglected in the same way that Negro quarters are frequently neglected in the American South. The municipality did nothing for the "coolie location," and then, perceiving the dangers to general health from this state of affairs, proceeded to destroy the "location" and dispossess the Indian settlers.

Gandhi was the lawyer for practically every Indian thus dispossessed. He tried some seventy cases and lost only one. The Indians involved, all illiterates, came to regard him as their greatest friend, and he was pleased beyond measure when they took to calling him *bhai* ("brother"). This remained his usual appellation in South Africa, and one he cherished beyond others—he never, in fact, reconciled himself to the word "*Ma-hatma*," and was only less hostile to the appellation *Bapu* ("Father"), which was universally used in his old age.

While he was in the midst of the litigation for the Indian quarters, there came an outbreak of the black plague —pneumonic plague, worse than bubonic. It arose in the gold-mining area, where the workers were mostly native African Negroes. But there were also Indians among them, of whom twenty-three came down with the plague one evening. The "coolie location" was overcrowded to a dangerous degree, and when Gandhi heard what had happened, he moved into the district at once, taking with him the four Indian boys who worked in his office. They

broke into an unoccupied house, transferred all the
plague patients there, and set up an improvised—and
quarantined—hospital, with Dr. William Godfrey as
their physician. In spite of the rapidity of the plague's
progress, they got all their patients through the night.

On the next day the municipality of Johannesburg
gave Gandhi an empty warehouse as a hospital for the
stricken Indians; the patients were all moved there. It
was usual to give brandy to plague patients at regular in-
tervals. Gandhi did not approve, and did not, in fact, believe that the brandy made any difference. He found
three patients willing to try his own methods of cure—
"earth and water" was his great discovery just then. To
these three he devoted himself, applying wet-earth poultices to their heads and chests through the critical period.
Two of the three lived. The third died—but so did all
the other twenty who were being treated with brandy.

The municipal nurse, a woman sent in on the second
day, was not allowed by Gandhi to touch the Indian patients for fear of giving her the contagion. Yet she got it
a day or so later and died in a very short time. Neither
Gandhi nor his four assistants, who were in close contact
with the patients, suffered any consequences at all. (This
strange immunity was to be repeated on numerous occasions throughout his life, when he nursed patients in
cholera, leprosy, and other eminently contagious dis-
eases.) Gandhi himself, although without any scientific
explanation for his immunity to contagion, tended to believe that it came in part from his extremely light diet in
times of such danger.

The Indian survivors (two) were moved to a plague
hospital seven miles from Johannesburg, and Gandhi's
emergency service came to an end.

It was just at this time, in the midst of the epidemic, that he acquired the devoted services of Mr. Albert West, an English vegetarian whom he had met in the diet restaurant they both frequented. Mr. West had a printing press, which gave Gandhi the idea that perhaps he would be willing to take charge of the *Indian Opinion* press at Durban. West agreed, and remained an invaluable co-worker for the whole time Gandhi was in South Africa.

Now the Johannesburg authorities decided that for the protection of the whole city the "coolie location," as a plague danger, would have to be burned to the ground. The Indian population was to be moved to tents in the great plain about thirteen miles away. Gandhi gave the municipality his full support in this project, and because the Indians, even against their will, were accustomed to following his advice, the deed was done without disturbance. The poor Indians were in a great fright, and as they (as illiterates) never had any dealings with a bank, they wanted to give all their savings to Gandhi. They had saved pennies and silver coins, mostly, and had buried them in the ground. It was now necessary to disinter their treasures and deliver them to their only friend, who accepted the trust with some misgivings. A very large sum, £60,000, came into his possession in this way. He gave a receipt for each sum, then had the coins disinfected and deposited them in his own bank. Later on he was able to persuade a good many of the Indians to convert these emergency deposits into permanent ones, so that the uses of the bank gradually made some headway. The day after the "coolie location" had been evacuated it was burned down by the police.

The Indians in their camp on the plains were merry again after a day's uncertainty; Gandhi rode out to see them every day on his bicycle, and it was his impression that the open air did them good.

5

Mr. West on arrival in Durban found that the affairs of *Indian Opinion* were not at all what Gandhi had understood them to be. The paper was not making a profit at all, as far as West could tell; but the bookkeeping had been done with such negligence that he could not be sure whether he was going to face a profit or a loss. Gandhi, startled at this, determined to go to Natal himself. On this journey from Johannesburg to Durban he read one of the most decisive books of his life, John Ruskin's *Unto This Last*. Gandhi read it with mounting excitement. He had at last found a text that was—to his always practical mind—practically a blueprint for what he most wished to do. Before he got off the train at Durban he was already resolved to put it into practice at once. Gandhi's own words on the *Unto This Last* occur in his autobiography, at the end of the eighteenth chapter.

I believe [he says] that I discovered some of my deepest convictions reflected in this great book of Ruskin, and that is why it so captured me and made me transform my life. A poet is one who can call forth the good latent in the human breast. Poets do not influence all alike, for everyone is not evolved in an equal measure.

The teachings of *Unto This Last* I understood to be:

1. That the good of the individual is contained in the good of all.

2. That a lawyer's work has the same value as the barber's, inasmuch as all have the same right of earning their livelihood from their work.

3. That a life of labor, i.e., the life of the tiller of the soil and the handicraftsman, is the life worth living.

The first of these I knew. The second I had dimly realized. The third had never occurred to me. *Unto This Last* made it as clear as daylight for me that the second and third were contained in the first. I arose with the dawn, ready to reduce these principles to practice.

Gandhi's peculiar mixture of idealism and practicality took from the book what he most needed, what most suited his inner nature—and, specifically, the idea of co-operative labor. As soon as he got off the train in Durban he told his loyal friend Mr. West that he wanted to move *Indian Opinion* to a farm—staff, presses, and all—where everybody would have a fixed work contribution and a fixed monetary allowance, equal for all. He hit upon three pounds per month as the sum that every person would receive, regardless of race or nationality. As there were about a dozen men involved in *Indian Opinion*, there was no unanimity in the matter; some wanted to stay in Durban; to some the idea of co-operative labor made no immediate appeal. To these Gandhi offered the chance to come in later if they liked the settlement.

Within two days he had arranged the matter and advertised for a tract of land near Durban. Within a week he had bought it—Phoenix, fourteen miles from Durban, was the railway station, and one hundred acres were for sale. Gandhi got the lot for one thousand pounds (backed in this, as in other "public work," by his friends among the Moslem merchants). Within a month he had built a big shed for the printing press, using volunteer labor from among Indian masons and carpenters who had been in his nursing corps during the Boer War, and materials supplied for nothing by the merchants.

From then on, *Indian Opinion* continued to be published at the Phoenix Settlement, which became the cen-

ter of Gandhi's activity in Natal. He tried to get some of
his relatives and followers to join the co-operative settlement, but a good many of them were making money in
business and did not relish the thought of giving it up.
One who did come and proved abundantly skillful as a
handicraftsman and ever loyal as a disciple was Maganlal
Gandhi, the second cousin who had come out from India
on the last trip.

The first issue of *Indian Opinion* from the settlement
was printed by hand because the oil engine refused to
work at the last minute. Gandhi mobilized not only his
own staff, but the Indian volunteer carpenters, and in re-
lays of four men throughout the night the press was
worked by a hand-wheel. We are entitled to suspect that
he rather enjoyed this victory of the human being over
the machine. Indeed, after some time, the settlement deliberately gave up the use of the oil engine and printed
the paper regularly by hand-wheel.

The land around the settlement was divided up into
plots of three acres each, and each member of the co-operative was responsible for the cultivation of his own
plot. Huts of corrugated iron were built, not because
they were wanted (Gandhi would have preferred
thatched cottages of mud or brick), but because they
were quick and cheap. Every member of the community
learned to set type and work the printing press, so that
there was a plentiful supply of labor for the paper. Gandhi describes himself as the dunce of the community so
far as typesetting was concerned, but his cousin Maganlal became a really expert compositor.

He was obliged to return to Johannesburg as soon as
the Phoenix Settlement had been well started. Through-

out these years, in fact, he had one foot in the Transvaal and one in Natal, a position difficult to maintain.

The hour of Gandhi's renunciation (his rather gradual renunciation) was at hand. No doubt the Zulu War, like everything else, had something to do with it, as did Ruskin, Tolstoy, Jesus, Buddha, and the Hindu Scriptures. The moment the Zulu "rebellion" broke out in Natal, Gandhi offered his services with an Indian ambulance corps, and to his astonishment, the Governor of Natal accepted at once (no doubt remembering the service given in the Boer War). In actual fact Gandhi's sympathies were with the Zulus, but he felt his loyalty to the British Empire to override everything else. He organized a corps of twenty-four Indian volunteers, who served through the Zulu War, and to his delight their task was to care for wounded or sick or injured Zulus.

Somehow the conflict set up in his mind by the Zulu War (his sympathy for the Natal natives and his loyalty to the Raj) worked itself out into a personal dilemma: brahmacharya. For some years he had been endeavoring, by every normal or ordinary means, to control his sexual appetites. Much of his dietary experimentation was related to this effort. Now he felt that the time had come to take the vow of chastity for the rest of his life. He discussed it with his co-workers and followers, many or most of whom were willing to take the vow with him. (His co-workers did not always fulfill their vows, but Gandhi never broke one in his life.) For Gandhi the vow meant not only chastity of the body, but purification of the mind, and he struggled for years to exclude from his conscious or unconscious mind every indication of bodily pleasure in sex. He was thirty-six (in the mid-

dle of 1906) when he took the vow irrevocably. As
years went on, in spite of the struggle, he became more
and more convinced that it was the only way to achieve
a selfless activity, a release of the spirit, and he found,
moreover, that his relationship with Kasturbai went into
a new and altogether different phase. His wife became
his most devoted friend and helper. The quarrels and
disturbances of other days faded away. It was by no
means easy, but he was persuaded that this "self-purification" was necessary not only for his own release, but also
for the birth of *satyagraha*, his distinctive creation, the
idea that changed the world.

Satyagraha had existed, of course, before he found a
name for it. His notions of sacrifice for the truth, voluntary abnegation and self-surrender in the service of the
community, challenge to the unrighteous law or to the
unjust application—all this, and all that relates to these
notions, had been growing in him for years past. It
needed to be made quite plain and clear so that every ordinary Indian person (unlettered, but willing to learn)
might absorb the idea and act upon it.

During this period, while he was absorbed in more
and rigorous dietary experiments (all designed to reduce
his physical lusts), Gandhi bethought himself of a way to
get a name for the qualities and purposes to which he had
decided to dedicate the Indian community in South Africa, himself first of all. He offered a small prize in *Indian Opinion* for a name that would crystallize his ideas
of the nature and method of struggle. His cousin Maganlal won the prize by suggesting the word *sadagraha*, from
sat (truth) and *agraha* (firmness or force), two Sanskrit
words that had not been combined in this way before.

Gandhi saw at once that this was the word, but it was

not quite plain enough for masses of Indians with no knowledge of Sanskrit. He therefore changed it to *satya* (a more comprehensible form) and *agraha*, making the word *satyagraha*. From then on, the word and the idea grew; they were to liberate India and put an end to the greatest of empires. The force of truth, the firmness of truth, the power of the soul—all these translations have been offered; all are better than the English expressions, such as "nonresistance" and the like, which had been used before.

6

Gandhi started another co-operative settlement later on near Johannesburg, as nearly as possible like the Phoenix Settlement, and called it the Tolstoy Farm. It was there (as much as at Phoenix) that many of his ideas evolved and were put into practice. Both the Tolstoy Farm and the Phoenix Settlement became flourishing establish-ments, with many men, women, and children living in each, and the experiments in education, vocational train-ing, diet, and discipline were ceaselessly interesting to Gandhi and fruitful for his subsequent creative activity. Much of the "Basic Education" system, now gaining ground rapidly throughout India, was developed by ac-tual work on the Tolstoy Farm and the Phoenix Settle-ment, Gandhi's own three younger boys being among the pupils. On one occasion, when a "moral lapse" (pre-sumably sexual) was discovered in the Phoenix com-munity, Gandhi abandoned all his public work and went from the Transvaal to Natal, where he fasted for seven days as a penance for the sin of the young people. His addiction to fasting as a form of penance, prayer, self-discipline, or purification was growing stronger every

year, but by this time it had already assumed a terrible
aspect to those who loved him—they lived in fear until
the fast was over, and many of them, in sheer terror and
repentance, fasted with him. This was true of Indians and
Europeans alike: in the case mentioned, his German
friend and follower Hermann Kallenbach fasted with
him day by day. Clearly the Gandhian influence and essence, so powerful that evidence to the contrary is quite
lacking, was becoming not only ethical (that it always
had been), but more and more irrational—in an ordinary sense, more and more religious. One could not assign definite reasons for anything he did, but whatever
he did—in obedience, more and more, to the "inner
voice" that spoke to him—had its effect.

The actual beginning of the *satyagraha* campaign in
South Africa may be dated from September 11, 1906.
(This year, the year of his final renunciation, was fateful
for Gandhi.) The government of the Transvaal had announced in the preceding month that it would introduce
a bill calling for the registration of all Indians above the
age of eight. They were to be finger-printed and were to
obtain certificates, which they must carry with them at
all times. They were to become an especially marked or
branded section of the population, with no doubt worse
to follow. If they disobeyed this ordinance, they were to
be imprisoned or deported or both.

In Johannesburg the Indian community called a mass
meeting at the Imperial Theatre, where, after a great deal
of indignation had been aired, the chairman called upon
all present to take a vow "with God as their witness."
This aroused Gandhi to a speech which—in spite of his
lingering shyness—was one of the greatest in his career.
He warned the three thousand persons present that they

must not call God to witness their vow unless they fully intended, literally and to the end, to carry it out. The vow was of disobedience to the law. He personally pledged himself "unto death," but warned all present that they must do the same or their vow would be meaningless. He injected such solemnity into the meeting that it grew hushed and tearful, but when the moment came to take the vow, every person present took it. He warned them that it might mean jail, hardship, cruelty, or death, and the preponderance of evidence is that his words were understood.

Gandhi himself appears to have had an ample realization of the magnitude of this vow. Before offering *satyagraha* (the voluntary sacrifice), which he must have known was an irresistible weapon, he decided to go to England to see if persuasion would do any good. He actually saw Lord Elgin, the Colonial Secretary (a former Viceroy of India), and John Morley, Secretary of State for India; they disapproved the proposed legislation, but only until the end of the year, when the Transvaal would cease to be a Crown Colony and become self-governing. The law was passed in due course and went into effect on July 31, 1907.

The Indians, most of them, stood firm, and although Gandhi's concept of *satyagraha* was not yet fully formed, and was far from being understood by his own followers, they understood one thing well enough, which was that they could not register under the iniquitous law and keep their self-respect. Among the first summoned before the magistrate for not doing so was Gandhi, who (January 11, 1908) asked the judge to give him the heaviest sentence, as he had deserved it. The judge gave him the lightest—two months of simple imprisonment, specify-

ing that it should be "without hard labor." It was Gandhi's first term in jail.

He seems almost to have enjoyed it. It was a holiday
from the oppressive and time-consuming work of all sorts
which had filled his days. He read the *Gita* in the morning and the *Koran* in the afternoon; he read Ruskin, Tolstoy, Bacon, and Plato; he taught English (by means of
the Bible) to a Chinese Christian who was a fellow prisoner. But his term was all too short: General Smuts
wanted to see him. The Chief of Police of Johannesburg
came to the jail and fetched Gandhi—in prison uniform
and without money or baggage—to Pretoria to see the
Prime Minister of the Transvaal.

General Smuts proposed a compromise by which the
Indians would voluntarily register; if they did so, the
objectionable act for compulsory registration would be
repealed. He spoke in a conciliatory tone to Gandhi, explaining that, whatever he personally thought of the law,
he could do nothing, as the European population over-
whelmingly demanded it. It is indeed probable that even
then Smuts had some personal sympathy for Gandhi, and
if so, it was reciprocated, for that was Gandhi's nature.
In any case, the compromise was made. Smuts told Gandhi he was free from that moment. When Gandhi asked
after the other Indian prisoners, Smuts said they would be
freed the following morning. Gandhi had no money and
had to borrow the fare to Johannesburg from Smuts's
secretary.

Smuts broke his word to Gandhi. After the latter had
persuaded many or most Indians to register voluntarily as
a compromise helpful to the government, Smuts proceeded to pass the Asiatic Act anyhow. Gandhi having
struggled very hard to persuade his fellow countrymen

to the compromise—and having indeed incurred a severe assault from some angry Pathans because he insisted
on being the first to register—this was a cruel blow. He
now had to mobilize his resources, such as they were, for
a more bitter and general struggle.

On August 16, 1908, at a mass meeting in Johannesburg, the Indian registrants—some two thousand of them
—burned their registration certificates in a caldron of
kerosene in the midst of great excitement. Under the Asiatic Act this rendered them all liable to imprisonment.

Volunteers, not on a mass basis as yet, but selected
with some care, were sent across the border from Natal
to the Transvaal without certificates. Among these was
Harilal, Gandhi's eldest son, who had now come from
India at last and joined the movement. Gandhi himself
defied the law and was arrested again on October 10,
1908.

During this second prison sentence Gandhi made another of his epochal literary discoveries: Thoreau. He
read Thoreau's essay (originally a lecture) called "Civil
Disobedience," concerned with his own refusal to support the American government (1849) because of slavery and the Mexican War. The essay is a fiery piece, and
contains many ideas upon which Gandhi had in fact
been acting for some years without knowing that they existed elsewhere. Now he absorbed these ideas, too, into
his Ruskin-Tolstoy edifice of authority. In jail, aside
from reading, Gandhi was cook to some seventy-five
other Indians. When volunteers were required for latrine duty, Gandhi volunteered.

The second prison sentence ended December 13,
1908, but upon his release he continued the *satyagraha*
movement and was quickly sentenced for a third term

(February 25, 1909). This time he went to the newly built penitentiary at Pretoria for a term of three months. He had borrowed his Thoreau from the jail library in Johannesburg; he seems to have found Emerson's essays in Pretoria, for we see in his letters that he was reading them and recommending them to his correspondents. It is a natural but very striking parabola, that by which Thoreau and Emerson, who owed so much to the *Gita* and the *Upanishads*, thus returned to India. The *Bhagavad-Gita* was in fact the only book of which Henry Thoreau died possessed. He kept it with him in his hut at Walden Pond; he valued it beyond "all the treasures of the east." Gandhi by now had memorized a large part of the *Gita* in Sanskrit; he used to paste it up, couplet by couplet, on his shaving mirror and learn it during the time of his morning ablutions. To find in far-off America —and by means of jail libraries in Africa—echoes of his beloved "song celestial" must have been a rare experience for Ghandi, for he referred to it repeatedly then and afterwards.

During this third jail sentence, General Smuts sent him two books, both of a religious nature.

When he was released this time, though the struggle against Indian disabilities continued, Gandhi resolved to try his luck at a higher court: he went to London and remained there from July to November 1909, ceaselessly talking, writing, and agitating for a hearing. His main reason for going was that the Union of South Africa was in process of being formed; Botha and Smuts had both gone to London; the danger was that the new Union might extend the Transvaal legislation to the whole country and brand the Indians forever. Gandhi by this time wanted some kind of general assurance of what he called "legal or theoretical equality in respect of immigration." If he could get that and remove the fundamental insult to Indian self-respect, the details could follow.

But Smuts, even under British pressure, was unwilling to go so far. Many elements in London deplored the anti-Indian legislation for a wide variety of reasons—some on ethical or religious grounds, some out of a sense of justice, and some because they felt it endangered Britain's imperial position in India. Gandhi was able to appeal to a very considerable number of Englishmen of influence. Smuts agreed, not too willingly, to repeal the objectionable Asiatic Act and to permit the immigration of selected Indians to the Transvaal—but they had to be hand-picked, limited in number, and all educated, English-speaking professionals of one sort or another (all Gandhis, in short). Anything like a concession of legal or theoretical equality he was quite unwilling (and possibly, in view of the feelings of his supporters, unable) to grant. The "badge of inferiority," as Gandhi called it, was to remain.

Gandhi returned to Africa at the end of the year with the consciousness that his struggle, now firmly called *satyagraha*, would have to be intensified. Those who followed his line of action—voluntary sacrifice is a better term for it in English than "civil disobedience" or "passive resistance"—were called *satyagrahis*. A *satyagrahi* had to struggle toward poverty, purity, abstinence, and restraint in order to be worthy to offer the sacrifice. Moreover, the problem of how to take care of a *satyagrahi*'s family and dependents while he was in jail had grown to some dimensions.

At this juncture Hermann Kallenbach, Gandhi's

sturdy German-Jewish friend and follower, bought a tract of land at a place called Lawley, twenty-one miles from Johannesburg, and presented it to Gandhi for the *satyagrahis*. It was a well-watered area of over one thousand acres, with orange, apricot, and plum trees. Gandhi formed another co-operative like the Phoenix Settlement, moved into it with his family, and called it the Tolstoy Farm. Here the *satyagrahi* could be at home when he was not in jail, and his family could stay when he was.

Gandhi's austerity, steadily on the increase, reached its permanent level on the Tolstoy Farm. There he took the vow not to drink cow's or buffalo's milk, having read that cruelty was used to increase their production. With his friend Kallenbach he embarked on a diet of fruit and nuts alone, with olive oil. Kallenbach, a rich or, at any rate, well-to-do man, shared every labor and dietary experiment, including the extremely early hours and the long walks Gandhi thought necessary for health.

The visit of Gokhale, Gandhi's "political guru," in the autumn of 1912 was a turning-point in the long struggle for Indian rights. Gokhale was highly respected both in India and in England: the South African government set itself out to give him a favorable impression. Gandhi accompanied him through most of his tour of the new Union, but did not go with him to see Botha and Smuts in Pretoria. The two Boer generals, now intent on the establishment of the Union without unnecessary difficulty, actually promised Gokhale that the worst of the Indian disabilities would be repealed. Gandhi was not prepared to believe this just yet, and he was right.

Smuts brought on the last battle by announcing that the European community in Natal refused to permit the

lifting of the poll tax. Natal had been the original creator of the system of Indian serfdom. Gandhi and his
family and friends moved at once to Natal—to Phoenix
Settlement—and prepared for the struggle. They were
vastly aided by a Supreme Court decision in the Cape
Colony declaring that only Christian marriages could be
valid in South Africa. This made all Indian wives con-
cubines, and their children bastards. It embittered the Indians more than anything that had gone before, and
aroused the women—hitherto not active in the movement—to a pitch of determination in sacrifice. *Satyagraha* was now to be enacted on a really large scale.

Gandhi decided that one group of women should offer sacrifice by crossing from the Transvaal to Natal without permission, while another group made the same offering by crossing from Natal to the Transvaal without
permission.

It was provided that if the "sisters" (as Gandhi called
them) from the Transvaal should not be arrested by the
Natal border police, they would go to the coal mines at
Newcastle and ask the indentured laborers to go on
strike. This was what took place: the Natal border police let the women go, and they brought on a strike of
five thousand coal miners at Newcastle. The Transvaal
police arrested the group from Natal and sent them to
jail for three months.

Gandhi betook himself to Newcastle, where he found
the miners determined to continue their strike and obey
his orders. He organized their camp, obtained food and
equipment for them from the Indian merchants, and then
debated what to do with them. They were his "army,"
and he could lead them all to jail if he wished. He talked
to them very seriously, urging them not to follow him

unless they were convinced that he was right, and depicting to them the hardships of jail in the Transvaal. When he found that not even one of them hesitated, he made his decision. They would all walk across the border into the Transvaal and go to jail for doing so.

His arrangements were careful, precise, and characteristic: every precaution of "hygiene and sanitation" was taken. His followers were not to struggle, must engage in no violence, and must not resist arrest, flogging, or other indignities at the hands of the police. He was himself in charge of cooking and sanitary rules. He notified the South African government (as was now his invariable custom and a part of *satyagraha*) that his "army" was about to march. After prayers on the morning of November 6, 1913, the march began.

At the first stop across the Transvaal border, Gandhi himself was arrested. Kallenbach had already arranged for his release on bail, so that he could go back to his "army," but on the next day he was arrested again, and again released on bail. Two days later it happened again, and this time there was no bail. His "army" had its orders, and was to continue to Tolstoy Farm or until arrested.

Gandhi, of course, pleaded guilty before the judge in Volksrust and asked for the maximum punishment, his unfailing practice in such cases. The judge obviously did not want to convict him and demanded evidence of his guilt. Two of Gandhi's best friends gave evidence against him, and he received a sentence of three months at hard labor. He then gave evidence against each of them in turn, and all three received the same sentence.

These arrests were accompanied and followed by large numbers of others. The "army" was arrested en

masse for deportation to Natal. New volunteers arose in
all parts of the country to court arrest. All of this, amply
reported in both England and India, stirred up a storm.

The "army," returned under guard to the coal mines
at Newcastle, refused, in spite of floggings and starvation, to go back to work. They were joined by others.
The strike movement spread with great rapidity until
fifty thousand indentured laborers (regarded as serfs in
the South African system) were refusing to do any work.
Thousands of free Indians, like Gandhi, were in jail.

The Viceroy of India (Lord Hardinge) demanded a
commission of inquiry, and the idea was taken up in
London. Botha and Smuts were faced with new difficulties. Their immediate solution was to release Gandhi,
with his friends Kallenbach and Polak, from prison (December 18, 1913). This was not at all what Gandhi
wished, for he could actually do more good in jail than
out. He seized his opportunity, just the same, attacked
the commission of inquiry as being a "packed" body hostile to the rights of the Indians, and announced that on
the first of the year (1914) he and a group of Indians
would march from Durban again to court arrest.

At this point the white employees of the South African
railroad system went on strike. There were messages of
solidarity, it seems, and perhaps the European white
workers felt that the Indians could help them; but Gandhi was against it. He called off his New Year's Day
march, explaining that *satyagraha* must be pure and must
not aim at humiliating or embittering the enemy. The
government was in great difficulties (it had in fact declared martial law): he would forbear.

Perhaps he gained more for the Indians by this forbearance than if he had pursued his intended course. In

any case, Smuts asked him to come to Pretoria and talk.
Friends had been arriving from England and India; the
Viceroy had sent a special emissary, Sir Benjamin Rob-
ertson, to defend the Indians.

The early months of 1914 were devoted to a long,
painstaking negotiation between Smuts and Gandhi.
There is little doubt that these two men acquired a high
regard for each other during their struggle; evidence is
abundant. "You can't put twenty thousand Indians into
jail," Smuts said, and indeed the jail system of South
Africa had already proved inadequate to the problem; he
was faced with a necessity. But aside from the strange
necessity created by *satyagraha,* he clearly came to regard
Gandhi with a respect bordering on awe and affection.

The agreement was finally made and expressed in an
exchange of letters (June 30, 1914) between the two.
It was legalized as the "Indian Relief Bill" and submitted
to the Union Parliament, in which it became law in July.
It declared Indian marriages (Hindu, Moslem, and Parsee) legal; it abolished the three-pound poll tax on indentured laborers, canceling all arrears; it declared that the
system of importing indentured laborers from India must
cease in 1920; and it provided that though Indians could
not leave one province for another without permission,
those born in South Africa might enter the Cape Colony.

Satyagraha had proved to be an irresistible weapon. It
was something so new at that time that it hardly seems to
have been comprehended either in India itself or in England. It was surrounded by Gandhi with such severe disciplines of self-control and non-violence that it represented something quite novel in the techniques of human
struggle. It was years before its full meaning could be
taken in by everybody in India and in England.

Gandhi's work in South Africa was now completed. On July 18, 1914, he sailed for England with Mrs. Gandhi and Mr. Kallenbach. Before he left, he asked his devoted friends Sonya Schlesin and Henry Polak to give Smuts a pair of sandals he had made in prison. These Smuts wore for twenty-five years, until Gandhi's seventieth birthday (1939), when he sent them to India as a token of friendship to their donor. "I have worn these sandals for many a summer since then," Smuts said then, "even though I may feel that I am not worthy to stand in the shoes of so great a man."

CHAPTER FOUR

INDIA—AND WAR

WHEN Gandhi left South Africa forever at the age of forty-five, he was already a fully formed personality. He had adopted practically all those disciplines with respect to diet, hours of work, exercise, meditation, prayer, and silence which were to be his unvarying rule thereafter. Some were not yet fixed—for example, the weekly day of silence had not come into being as an unalterable rule just yet. But all the elements were there. One conspicuous exception was the clothing: he still wore English clothes, though he had already appeared at several public meetings in South Africa in Indian clothing. He had not yet found the spinning-wheel, but it was already in his mind, and he only awaited his return to India to set about finding it. He was ready for India. It was not in his naturally modest mind to suppose that India was ready for him, too, but he found that out in due course.

The great achievements of *satya, ahimsa, brahmacharya* (truth, non-violence, and self-control or chastity) had been made. He had probably been rigidly truthful for a good many years, but was to refine and purify his views of truth for the rest of his life. *Ahimsa*, the forbearance and respect for all life which are deeply engrained in Hinduism, had been native to him from birth; he was steadily amplifying it so that it came to be, finally, something like what the Christians call "love" or "charity." That is, it was not simply non-violence, an absence of violence, but a positive extension of the hand to every form of life. And *brahmacharya*, which the Hindu sages regarded as essential for all students and all sages (that is, at the two extremes of the ages of man), had been his since his thirty-sixth year, though not easily or without pain.

His external success in leading the Indians of South Africa to victory in their human rights was to a very considerable degree the result of his self-conquest in these matters. He felt, probably quite correctly, that he could not lead unless he was himself pure. It has been said innumerable times that nobody can really lead India without first "renouncing the world." Gandhi's renunciation was gradual, and he apparently still paid his own expenses out of funds acquired by professional activity; but by the age of forty-five he had already gone a very long way on the road. He not only had given up sex and the pleasures of food, as well as any gain not strictly necessary for life, but also had surrendered savings, life insurance, possessions of all sorts (including his wife's jewelry) and all aspects of social consideration except those necessary for the self-respect of the Indian community. He had very little more to do to become an embodiment of renunciation. The eternal puzzle as to whether so mighty a power—and his was the mightiest of his time—belongs to a *sannyasin*, one who has renounced the world, can never really be settled. In this matter the extremes really do meet, and very dramatically. We see in him a man of no possessions or appetites, a true *sannyasin*, and yet from the depths of his renunciation he dictates to empires and models the course of history. It may be a paradox, but in ordinary, simple fact it happened in plain view of the whole modern world, and therefore cannot be contested.

He was small, gentle, sad, with mournful eyes, and

with ears that stuck out at right angles, as always. His physical endurance was fantastic—sometimes he used to walk from Tolstoy Farm to Johannesburg and back on the same day, roughly fifty miles, to save money—and yet it was sustained on the slightest diet possible. At that time it consisted merely of fruits and nuts, with no milk at all and no vegetables. He had already taken up the habit of fasting as a form of prayer, and giving fixed limits (in the form of vows) to his fasts. He would vow, for example, to fast for seven days in atonement for a sin committed by some of his followers. Nothing could prevent the fulfillment of the vow. At other times (and still more, later) he would fix no limit, but fast simply until he felt that the "inner voice" permitted him to cease. These great fasts were conceived and executed as prayers to God, either in atonement or in aspiration, but in later days, when so many governments were forced to yield on so many points because of them, they came to seem a form of political pressure, and indeed from an external point of view they resembled such a process. Only when they are considered as a logical development of his own life (beginning in South Africa, where no fast had any effect on public events) can we see how necessary they were to him.

The chief concomitant of *satyagraha*, as Gandhi developed it in South Africa and on a much greater scale later in India, was loyalty to the opponent. You must tell your opponent what you are going to do, precisely and without the faintest deviation from fact. You must accept his course of action, which you yourself have foreseen and chosen. (Asking the maximum penalty was a form of this.) You must never deceive your opponent or take unfair advantage of him. He must always be aware to the full of what you intend. He is, in fact, your friend, from whom you are temporarily separated by a disagreement, but you must never forget that he is your friend. These precepts were fully in effect (and practically too, by experience) before Gandhi returned to India. They probably account for the circumstance, so often noted, that many of his opponents—jailers, policemen, detectives, jail doctors, and the like—became his greatest friends.

2

The First World War broke out two days before Gandhi landed in England from South Africa. He immediately set about the formation of an Indian ambulance corps for the British army. He believed that because he accepted all the benefits of British rule, he had some obligation toward that rule. His loyalty, which had never flinched and was not to suffer any change for another five years, was clear and plain. He was a subject of the British Empire, and although, like members of some other religious sects (such as the Quakers) he was unable to perform acts of violence in its defense, he was still loyal and would do what he could within his bounds. He even realized, and said, that working in an ambulance corps was philosophically the same as taking part in the violence of war. Even so, it was what his religious conscience permitted.

But he fell ill after a few weeks—this time it was pleurisy—and after some experiments with diet he accepted the doctor's advice and went home to India. To his sorrow, his friend Kallenbach, a German, was not

allowed to go with him: even the Viceroy of India (Lord
Hardinge) was unwilling "to take the risk" of giving
him a visa.

The return to India was in many respects a great surprise to Gandhi. He had been away most of twenty
years, with part of his mind always intent upon India,
but with most of his time and energy given to the special
problem of the Indians in South Africa. He could hardly
have expected to be greeted by great crowds in the streets
of Bombay (January 9, 1915). His previous visits home
had produced no excitement of the sort. But in the meantime he had been victorious in his South African struggle; the new weapon of *satyagraha* had been forged and
put to uses unknown; and he himself had become Mahatma ("Great Soul") to large numbers of people.

In India at the time of his death and at other times I
have been at pains to inquire how this title or appellation
came to be given to him. I never could find anybody who
could fix a date for it. It unquestionably started in India,
among those who were watching his South African struggle from afar during the years before 1914. The appellation is not uncommon in India, or was not uncommon
until Gandhi came along. There have been other Mahatmas in the twentieth century, for example, whom nobody
today remembers. Once it got itself fastened upon Gandhi firmly, and by the usage of hundreds of millions of
people, it became almost like a part of his name, and it
may never be used for anybody else in the future.

Arising as it does from the people, however, and without any given source or authority, such a title is almost
impossible to trace down. Rabindranath Tagore ad-
dressed Gandhi as "Mahatma" in 1916 in a telegram
that has been preserved; he is supposed to have referred

to him as "Mahatma" before that. But it cannot be said that Tagore invented or bestowed the appellation. Sarojini Naidu was one of Gandhi's oldest friends and followers. She met him first in London in 1914, before his return to India, when he was living in a lodging-house in Bloomsbury. At that time he was already called "Mahatma," and Mrs. Naidu, in telling me this, could not remember for how long she had already heard him called by that name. Mr. Nehru met him first in 1916, and distinctly remembers that he had been "Mahatma" already for years before their meeting.

It seems simply to have exhaled from the people during his absence from India, and when he went home again he was already the "Great Soul." He did not actually like it. He refused to believe that there could be "greater" or "smaller" souls, and the reverence surrounding a Mahatma was a nuisance to him in the prosecution of his severely practical work. No doubt it was also an immense advantage, in a country like India, to have such an aura, and indeed his work could not have been done without it, but when it made him unable to walk through a crowd or get to a given destination, he grew impatient. Through many long years he learned to endure it, and with it the pitiless attention of the entire country to every deed of his life—and the crowds, the unbelievable Indian crowds!—but the evidence is that he never really accepted either the appellation or its significance.

3

The Mahatma's first year at home was spent, at the request of his revered "political guru," Gokhale, in retirement from public life. Gokhale felt that this strangely powerful little man was an instrument of India's destiny, but wisely saw that he required time to soak in the Indian air again, to grow familiar with the country and the life of the people.

Immediately after Gandhi's landing at Bombay on January 9, 1915, he was interviewed by the Governor of Bombay, Lord Willingdon, afterwards Viceroy of India, whom many remember as a man almost as gentle, in his way, as Gandhi himself. Willingdon asked him to promise that in the event he should wish to take steps concerning the government he would give notice first— the expression was: "Come and see me." Gandhi had not the slightest difficulty giving such a promise.

The "family" from South Africa, those who lived on Tolstoy Farm and in the Phoenix Settlement, had taken all the Gandhi vows and were real *satyagrahis*, needed to be reassembled in India. Most of them had been sent direct to India by Gandhi and had been cared for at Shantiniketan, in Bengal, the school and settlement (still in existence) of Rabindranath Tagore. The Mahatma now wanted to find a home of his own for this fairly numerous "family." He found it, eventually, in the neighborhood of Ahmedabad, the textile-manufacturing town that was the capital of his native Gujarat province. The Society of the Friends of India supplied the money necessary for the purchase of the land and the building of the huts. Gandhi hoped that the rich merchants of Ahmedabad, his fellow Gujarati, would provide the funds to continue the work, and for some time they did.

But before he opened his settlement and school—the Indian word for such a settlement is *ashram*—two events of some importance occurred. First came his visit to Shantiniketan, to Tagore, to see Tagore's *ashram* and visit his own twenty-five or more followers harbored there. Tagore's *ashram* consisted of about one hundred and twenty-five Bengali boys and a score of teachers. Gandhi's *ashram*, men, women, and children, belonged to several castes, sects, races, and religions. It included two Englishmen, Winstanley Pearson and "Charlie" Andrews, his devoted followers. The difference between the two *ashrams* was like the difference between Tagore and Gandhi themselves—the Poet, as he was called, remote and beautiful and sonorous and rich; the Mahatma small, busy, earnest, humble, and penniless. Gandhi at Shantiniketan did not like the use of hired servants to do the work, and with Tagore's permission he initiated a system of self-help in which the boys (all students of poetry and philosophy) learned to do everything, including the work of untouchables. The enthusiasm lapsed after Gandhi's departure, and Shantiniketan returned to the system of hired servants.

For he was called away, back to the other side of India, by the death of his "sure guide," Gokhale. This, though anticipated, was a great grief to him, and it is quite likely that it made him feel even more insecure during his first year in India. His position was peculiar. All the political classes in India were highly aware of him; in many sections of the masses he was extremely well known for his work in Africa; yet he was himself unknown to most of them. He could travel almost anywhere, in the most crowded third-class compartments, without being recognized by strangers. He had not spoken publicly or to any large audience. That personal attachment which Indians in general were to feel for him for so many long years was still in the future.

And the probability is that he was not himself sure of

what to do. He was quite content to build his *ashram*, take care of family, school, and communal work, remain silent on public questions, and study his surroundings. He thought, he tells us, that it might be five years or more before any opportunity would arise for the use of *satya-graha* in India. He had proved that soul-force was a great power, but he did not know how it would be applied in the service of India. It seems most likely that he did not anticipate its use in a political struggle, but he was well aware that it was a great discovery and as such was bound in time to be useful to India.

The *ashram*—it was called the *Satyagraha Ashram*, but came to be known before long, from the place where it was built, as Sabarmati—was founded May 25, 1915. Sabarmati was near enough to Ahmedabad to bear a close relation to it, far enough away to be independent of it in daily life. In the original *ashram* there were some twenty-five persons all vowed to chastity, poverty, and a life of service, all committed to every form of communal work, including that usually performed by untouchables (scavenging in particular, upon which Gandhi insisted). Not long after he had opened the *ashram*, he admitted a family of untouchables.

As the kitchens and water-supply and everything else in Gandhi's settlement operated by co-operative labor, the admission of a man, wife, and child from the untouchable outcastes was a revolutionary thing in India. At that time, and to this very day for many caste Hindus, the accidental touch of an untouchable implies pollution and certain purifying rites must be performed. Even the *shadow* of an untouchable pollutes. Any well used by untouchables is polluted and may not be used by caste

Hindus. Untouchable servants in the house may do certain tasks and no others. Those tasks (the dirtiest ones,
of course) may not be performed by servants of the
higher castes.

There were no servants in Gandhi's *ashram*. All were
equal and all shared in the same work for the same pay,
although of course some were better at some things than
at others. The Mahatma himself was never very expert,
as we have seen, as a compositor, but he worked faith-
fully at printing just the same in times of stress, to do his
part. He became in time a superb spinner and weaver,
but he always admitted that his second cousin Maganlal
was better at both (as he was in typesetting also).

What he could do, and with surprising energy for
such a small and apparently frail man, was manual labor,
including the digging of latrines and the transport of ex-
crement. This is the lowest labor known to India, and
can be performed only by untouchables. His own performance of such tasks was forgiven by everybody, practically from the start, because "holy men" for thousands
of years have been like that—humble, willing to do all
work. This is an Indian tradition as old as any other. It
is for this reason that "holy men" (*sadhu*) are supposed
to be completely outside the caste system—they are too
erratic to obey the rules of caste.

But real, living untouchables, actual members of a
pariah classification, were a different matter. The moment
Gandhi admitted some real untouchables to his *ashram*
he was in trouble, because this meant that caste Hindus
were cooking and eating with pariahs, drinking the same
water and living an equal life with them. By doing the
work of untouchables Gandhi did not offend the caste

system too deeply; he was a "Great Soul" and could do it; but by admitting untouchables to equality with all others he offended his contemporaries to the depths.

Consequently all his income was cut off. He did not have much—it was a frugal *ashram* indeed, and aimed at becoming self-supporting—but such as he had came by the gift of the neighboring rich, all caste Hindus. They were incensed at him. The storm spread, and Indian opinion everywhere was aroused against him.

In this emergency he quite calmly decided upon his course: he and all his family and followers would move into the untouchable quarter of the city, would do untouchable labor, and would themselves become untouchables. Such a thing, if it had happened, would have shaken India far more than anything yet. But it did not happen. The usual Gandhi miracle occurred—a man unknown to him, a Moslem, appeared from nowhere and gave him a purse of rupees sufficient to sustain his *ashram* for an entire year. By the time the year was over, the storm had subsided, and even perfectly orthodox Hindus were willing to contribute to the support of Gandhi's work, as they continued to do throughout his life, even though his practice of absolute equality must have aroused their deepest prejudices.

The untouchable family who came to Gandhi then (1915) were Dudabhai (the man, a former teacher in the Bombay schools for untouchables), his wife, Danibehn, and their small daughter, Lakshmi, whom Gandhi afterwards adopted.

This episode, which may seem small, in retrospect, was not small at the time. It was discussed with excitement all over India. Almost every Indian leader of renown for generations past had denounced untouchability

as a distortion of the caste system. The greatest animators
of the spiritual renaissance at the end of the nineteenth
century, such as Ramakrishna, had opposed it with elo-
quence. Most of these men were Brahmins, and certainly
all were caste Hindus. Not one had ever thought of
bringing an untouchable into the house as an equal, sharing food and drink, dining at the same table. It must be
remembered that at this period high-caste Hindus did not
dine with members of castes other than their own, either
higher or lower. It was not done. Nobody had ever
heard of dining with an untouchable. Theory was one
thing; practice another. Many great Hindus had denounced the abuses of the caste system. Gandhi, who had
also denounced them and continued to do so, took the
significant further step of ignoring them altogether. From
this time onward it was understood in India that he meant
what he said.

4

Gandhi's year of silence came to an end at the opening ceremonies of the Hindu University at Benares,
where he spoke on February 4, 1916. The university,
now a heavily endowed institution with many modern
buildings, had grown from very slight beginnings some
twenty-odd years before, the original founder being Annie Besant. After the grand opening ceremonies of the
new university, to which fortunes had been given by
maharajahs and other rich Hindus, Mrs. Besant presided
over a meeting where Gandhi spoke. It was his declaration of personal independence, his profession of faith and
introduction to method. The students, professors, maharajahs, and British officials who listened to him must have
felt obscurely that something new had occurred, because

they received him very frostily. He was actually not allowed to finish. When cries of "Sit down, Gandhi!" began to be heard, Mrs. Besant, who was no doubt the
most scandalized of all, ordered the Mahatma to stop
speaking. He, of course, submitted.

What he had to offer was a criticism of India, of the
opening ceremonies of the university, of the Indian
princes, of the pomp and ceremony, the jewels and the
fanfares, while most of India starved in dirt, and untouchability was rampant. In his gentle, modest, slow,
and thoughtful way, Gandhi was always critical, because
in fact he had a supremely critical intelligence, but on this
occasion he seems to have been almost exclusively so. He
began by saying that he regretted the necessity for speaking in a foreign tongue (English) at the opening of a
Hindu national university. He spoke then of self-government, and of the necessity for action rather than speeches.
He said self-government could not come by the efforts
of the lawyers, journalists, landlords, and the like, but
only through the masses of the people. He made severe
references to the jewels seen the day before on the hats,
collars, and bosoms of the Indian princes, and to the general extravagance of the ceremonies. He spoke of Indian
lack of sanitation, of the intolerable conditions in third-
class carriages on the railway trains, of spitting, and of
other things most unpleasant for his upper-class Indian
audience to hear. On such festal occasions in particular,
Indians do not like to be reminded of their shortcomings.
Many notables left the meeting, and finally the disorder
grew to be uncontrollable by Mrs. Besant, or so she
thought, and she adjourned the meeting. Gandhi had, in
his way, thrown down the gauntlet.

The attack upon Indian conditions was thoroughly in

Gandhi's character. That was how he had begun in South Africa, too—by telling the Indians what they ought to do to make themselves better, more self-respecting, and therefore more respected. Emphasis on sanitation, education, good conduct, and common sense was nothing new to him: he had followed this exact line for twenty years of public work in South Africa, and it had borne remarkable results. It was, however, quite new in India. The fashion in India then, as now, was to tell the Indians how remarkable was their culture, how ancient their tradition, how noble their aim. Mrs. Besant, for instance (then about seventy), had been stamping up and down all India for years past lecturing the Indians about the glories of their philosophical origin. She had done a superb kind of resurrection, in a way, because many of the young men who listened to her (and they were all of the privileged classes, because she spoke only in English) had never really thought much about their cultural heritage until she, an Englishwoman, came along to tell them. But even Mrs. Besant, with her great love for India, was incapable of realizing how Mahatma Gandhi could upbraid his compatriots on such a solemn occasion, as a prelude to asking them for something better.

The opening of the Hindu University was in a simple chronological sense the beginning of Mahatma Gandhi's public life in India. The speech was repeated throughout the country, mostly, in those pre-radio days, by word of mouth, and lost nothing in the telling. It came to seem that a holy man, living like the poor, had spoken for the poor as against the rich. He had not spoken against the British at all—merely as an Indian among Indians, talking about India. The echoes were heard from the Himalayas to Cape Cormorin.

The first results of Gandhi's emergence were an increase of demands upon his time: requests to speak, to
espouse a cause, to help a group of struggling Indians.
He had much to do at his *ashram*, was busy writing at the
time, and was already engaged in the search for the spinning-wheel, but he did as much as he could to satisfy
these demands. The real opportunity—the Gandhian opportunity, to accomplish a suitable task in a characteristic
way—arose more or less by accident, as such oppor-
tunities always did. An obstinate peasant sharecropper
named Shukla turned up at the annual convention of the
Indian National Congress at Lucknow in December
1916, that very same at which Gandhi and Nehru met
for the first time and were not greatly impressed. The
peasant Shukla would not take no for an answer; he
wanted the Mahatma to come to his district, Champaran,
and see how abominably the indigo-cultivators were being
treated. The Mahatma had no time. Shukla waited—and
not only waited, but followed the Mahatma wherever he
went, even to the *ashram*, and there remained for weeks
on end.

Finally Gandhi went to Champaran. His reluctance
to do so had been partly due to the fact that he was very
busy on a subject near his heart: the abolition of indentured emigration from India—that is, of labor bound by
contract to South Africa—for which he asked general
Indian support and government approval. He fixed the
date for the abolition of such emigration as May 31,
1917: he had already found that words like "eventually"
and "in due course" were subject to much elasticity of
interpretation. The government abolished indentured emigration before the date he had named.

In the Champaran district Gandhi undertook a form

of action peculiarly his own, and related psychologically to much that became almost a pattern thereafter. He started in Patna, the capital of Bihar province, where a considerable number of lawyers and Congress members and other middle-class Indians had some sympathy for the sharecroppers and had (for fees) undertaken some of their court cases.

The Mahatma asked these men to go with him to the Champaran district, in the upper part of the province, and give their services, either in full or part-time, for nothing. From such volunteers he expected a good deal: they must be willing to go to jail, if necessary. They must pledge these things explicitly before setting forth. The system was new, and it took a little time for Gandhi to win over a sufficient number of fellow workers.

The next step was to warn the opponent (in this case the head of the indigo-planters' association and the government commissioner for the district) that he intended to investigate the grievances. From the tone of their response he knew that there would be trouble and in all probability jail for him. He proceeded just the same, in an orderly manner, with the taking of depositions from indigo sharecroppers as they came to him.

The situation was novel in the extreme. Gandhi had no official rank or standing of any kind—indeed, no right, as the angry planters declared, to be in Champaran at all. And yet his personality attracted such throngs of the downtrodden indigo-workers that it was quite impossible to flog them for obeying his summons. In the dilemma the local magistrate decided to order Gandhi out of the district, and when the Mahatma politely refused to go, he was summoned to stand trial the next day. The magistrate was taken aback by Gandhi's attitude, then so new as to be unknown in India: the Mahatma simply declared that he was guilty as charged and asked for the legal punishment. This was his course ever afterwards. Judgment was postponed, and in the meantime the Government of India, somewhat disturbed over the wide attention given to these events, ordered the case withdrawn.

Gandhi then proceeded with his depositions. So many thousands of them were unnecessary, but he had realized from the start that these desperately poor indigo-workers, accustomed to starvation and floggings, needed above all things to be "free from fear," as he said. Therefore, to give them the sense of having a friend, to free them from the fears of the defenseless, he encouraged them all to tell their stories and he listened to all with equal patience. It required from five to seven of the volunteers from Patna to be on duty all the time to take down the depositions, or full notes on them, as they were given.

In the meantime, as usual, Gandhi was also busy with dietary and sanitary problems. His volunteers from Patna, being lawyers and others in good circumstances, had their own cooks and body-servants; they had their meals separately at all hours, and were still highly unfamiliar with Gandhi's ways. It took him some time to induce them to have all their meals together from a common commissary and to have these meals exclusively vegetarian.

Furthermore, the villages of the indigo-workers were squalid with filth and vulnerable to every disease. Gandhi began his customary scavenging, washing, sweeping, and cleaning, with six villages chosen to start the operation. He had to get volunteers from other parts of India to do this work, much of which could normally be done only by untouchables if done at all. He started village schools in these six spots, and hoped that the example, even if it only lasted for a few months, would make some difference.

And in all this work, of course, the usual detective from the Criminal Investigation Department was beside him, noting all down and making reports. These C.I.D. detectives accompanied Gandhi wherever he went and whatever he did for about thirty years, and he invariably treated them with great courtesy. In the result some became his devoted friends.

At length the government grew weary of the campaign in Champaran, which had by now drawn the attention of all India. Inquiry was made when Gandhi would leave the district: he replied that he would do so when the grievances of these oppressed sharecroppers were recognized as being real and deserving of action. The government set up a commission of inquiry, with Gandhi as a member, and as a result the system by which three twentieths of the land had to be worked in indigo for the benefit of the landlord was abolished by law.

The Champaran experience may be called the first triumph of *satyagraha* in India, even though the *satyagraha* involved was for the most part Gandhi's alone. He had gained an objective of importance to human welfare, and had done so by his own distinctive means of truth, self-control, and non-violence, but his methods had still been most imperfectly understood even by those who applied them. He had to spend hours a day in explaining, even to his own volunteers, what these principles were and why they were necessary. Some volunteers wanted to accept money from the poor peasants, which Gandhi would never permit; whatever money was needed for the work had to come by gift from the privileged, mostly well-to-do people in Patna. The rigid rule of truth was another difficulty, for a certain amount of imagination is always rife in India as in other countries, and a story seldom loses in retelling. The Mahatma's insistence on literal, exact truth was difficult and even downright mysterious to many people for years afterwards. It seemed to him, all through these years, the center of his system, related to his general doctrine of means and ends. The means must be harmonious with the ends: good ends cannot be obtained by bad means. The truth must therefore rule all along the line, and any deviation from it will impair the purity of the *satyagraha*. These were difficult notions to introduce to the middle-class Indians who were his volunteers, for they had spent their lives taking full advantage (sometimes or often unconsciously) of their own advantages. That they accepted such disciplines, whether with comprehension or not, speaks eloquently for the persuasive power of Gandhi's personality.

5

Champaran was, in practical action, the introduction of *satyagraha* to India. It was soon followed by the introduction of another characteristic peculiarity of the Mahatma's genius—a fast for a specific purpose.

No part of the Gandhian system has been more discussed than the fast. To many persons of all countries it has seemed that this was a distinct weapon of political or social struggle, and that it had an essentially violent nature though the violence was done to the Mahatma himself rather than to others. There were times when Gandhi's opponents contended that his fasts were, in objective fact, little more than a kind of blackmail.

It is true that very important results often followed his fasts. It is also true that they were, at times, so specific in their purposes that they had every appearance, to the un-thinking, of a species of coercion.

As against this view the principal facts to be cited are: first and most of all, that fasting as a form of prayer was deep in Gandhi's psychological structure and was en-twined with his earliest memories; second, that he took this punishment upon himself, but never wished to extend it to others; third, that he had already fasted a great many times, in prayer for various purposes, or in atonement for various actions by his own followers, before the world in general paid any great attention; and last, that he tried hard, when impelled to fast (and often by his "inner voice"), to avoid giving this form of prayer the aspect of coercion upon others.

There can hardly be room for doubt that fasting was as natural to Gandhi as feasting might be to men of an-other kind. He had fasted all his life. His capacity to do so was phenomenal, and although in the extremely long fasts he underwent great agonies, he always maintained that a brief fast was salutary to body and mind. It seems to be true that he emerged from many of his fasts rein-vigorated for his struggle. The lightness of body and clarity of mind induced by a short fast may be experi-enced by anybody, quite without special preparation or training for it. Gandhi's peculiarity, physically, was a capacity to prolong his fasts to great lengths without suf-fering any great permanent injury.

Moreover, it can be maintained that the general nature of every fast he undertook in India was that of a prayer for peace. The specific purposes were various; their gen-eral character as prayer was for peace between factions in religion, race, and caste or in situations that threatened violence. Some fasts were in atonement for violence committed by Gandhi's own followers, and these, too, can be classified in the same general way as prayers for peace. The terrifying power these fasts exercised later, when practically all business ceased throughout the subcontinent, and governments scurried to find a way of bringing the ordeal to an end, could hardly have been foreseen in 1917. And yet in 1917, at the time of this first declared fast in India, Gandhi was already a completely formed character, in whom the fast as a form of prayer had long since entered as a permanent element.

The fast took place as a result of responsibilities he had assumed toward the millworkers of Ahmedabad, who had come to him for advice. These were his own people, of course, to whom he talked in his native Gujarati. Their employers, the millowners, were also his friends, and a good many of them had contributed to the upkeep of his *ashram*. Upon investigating, and talking to both sides, Gandhi decided that the mill-hands' grievances were legitimate and that the millowners were unwilling to give any satisfaction. Therefore he advised the mill-hands to go on strike, but only on condition that they would pledge themselves to total non-violence. They were to earn their daily bread in some way outside the mills, but not to take any action (such as toward strike-breakers) which could be called violent.

The mill-hands took this vow, at his request, and continued to take it daily for the next two weeks, coming out from the city to the *ashram* by the river to renew it. This established his own feeling of responsibility for them. With time the zeal for non-violence declined, and there was grave danger of attacks on strike-breakers. At this point the Mahatma, much troubled, decided to fast until the mill-hands returned to their vow of non-violence to the end. The fast lasted "only three days," Gandhi said. After that time the employers and workers had a meeting, decided on arbitration, and settled the strike.

The Ahmedabad fast has troubled even some of Gandhi's followers because it was so specific that it looked like a threat. This he never intended, but his intentions were sometimes difficult to make clear to persons whose whole preparation was unlike his own. In objective fact the fast brought the strike to an end, but its purpose was that of a prayer to hold the mill-hands (for whom he accepted responsibility) to their vow of non-violence. The distinction is important for any understanding of the nature of Gandhi's fasts, which were to play such a great part in the subsequent evolution of the Indian story.

"I fasted to reform those who loved me," was Gandhi's way of stating it: that is, to keep the mill-hands to their vow of non-violence. Settlement of the strike was the result, not the intention.

6

The end of Gandhi's life as a loyal subject of the British Empire was now not long in the future. As a final expression of this loyalty, which he had felt and expressed from childhood, he undertook to recruit soldiers for the (British) Indian Army during the summer of 1918.

The episode was so uncharacteristic that it disquieted his friends and admirers at the time, and has puzzled many since. His views, though stated often enough, were not understood. He had been loyal during the Boer War and the Zulu War, and in 1914, in each case providing the combatants with an Indian ambulance corps. He was de-voted to non-violence, and yet, as he had always accepted British protection, he felt that he should give what help

he could to sustain it. He did so, however, in the full
expectation that his effort—and India's—would be re-
warded by a "share in the partnership" of empire, which
is to say, in the language of 1918, by home rule. He
further asked the Viceroy (Lord Chelmsford) to ask the
London government to make some provision for the restoration of the Moslem Caliphate, destroyed by the defeat
of Turkey. He did not bargain with the Viceroy or anybody else, since this was against his principles in a matter
of conscience: he merely said, in a letter published
throughout India, what his hopes were, and told the
Viceroy that "disappointment of hope means disillusion."

He then embarked on a long, arduous tramp from village to village in the Kheda district of his native Gujarat
country, trying to enlist men for the army. This was a
district in which he had engaged in a *satyagraha* campaign
only a short time before in aid of the poor peasants who
were being sold up for tax arrears after a crop failure.
The Kheda campaign had brought him the support of all
the villagers, though *satyagraha* was imperfectly understood then and required hours a day of patient explanation. It had ended with a partial victory, the government
agreeing to remit taxes for the very poor if the richer
peasants (equally hard hit by crop failure) paid.

Gandhi had not been very pleased with the *satyagraha*
campaign in the Kheda district; too much money had
been spent on it by rich Bombay sympathizers, for one
thing, and there was too much hullabaloo in the press. Its
results did not please him either. But during the campaign he had felt the full, warmhearted support of the
country people.

Now it was a grievous disappointment and shock to
him to find that when he went among them as a recruiting

agent for the army, he was greeted with cold incompre-
hension and even hostility. "What about non-violence?
How can you ask us to take up arms? What good has
this government ever done to India?" Questions like
these were fired at him in village after village. They
would perhaps not have impressed themselves so deeply
on his consciousness if they had not found echoes in its
depths. He himself had asked the same questions before
he had undertaken the incongruous task. Now he re-
doubled his efforts, wore his body to a shadow, worried
and fretted over his lack of response, his inability to make
the people understand his point of view. In the result he
succumbed to a severe attack of dysentery, his first serious
illness.

He was not a good patient: he refused medicines and
almost any form of treatment the doctors could devise.
He fasted; he refused to change his nuts-and-fruit diet
even when he was willing to eat; his body was diminish-
ing at a startling rate. He would not eat eggs in any form,
and the doctors ran into the difficulty of the vow when
they recommended milk. At this point Kasturbai, his
patient wife, had the final say. "Your vow was against
cow's milk or buffalo's milk," she said. "It did not include
goat's milk."

(Two days before his death he described the scene for
me. "I can see her now," he said, and there is not much
doubt that it was she who found the solution, in alliance
with his own will to live.)

He accepted goat's milk and lived. Thereafter he continued to drink goat's milk, though it worried him that
he might be breaking the spirit of his vow in honoring
the letter. The implication (in his account to me) was
that in 1912 he would have vowed not to drink goat's

milk either if he had thought of it, but since he had not
thought of it, it was not included. The "weakness of the
flesh" was responsible for his drinking goat's milk until
the end. There seems little doubt that it provided a necessity without which he could not have continued existence.

During this illness a message arrived from the Viceroy
saying it was no longer necessary to recruit soldiers: Ger-
many had surrendered. This relief from a task he must
have disliked intensely may have contributed to Gandhi's
recovery, which was very slow, but steady. He was very
weak for months after the bout of dysentery, and during
those months engaged in no public work, aside from work
in his own *ashram*.

During this winter after the war, the report of the
Rowlatt Committee was published and the convalescent
Gandhi read it. The Rowlatt Committee had been appointed as a committee of inquiry to study Indian sedition and how to deal with it. Its report recommended an
extension into peacetime of all the wartime rigors in suppression of free speech, freedom of the press, and the
right of assembly.

Gandhi, too feeble to act at once, studied the document with mounting indignation. If this was India's re-
ward in time of peace, what hope could there be for home
rule? Against the protests of all Indian leaders, the principles of the Rowlatt report were embodied in a law that
the government of India sent to the Legislative Council
(made up largely of English officials) early in 1919.
The ailing Gandhi dragged his feeble frame to Delhi and
listened to the debate. It ended, as had been foreseen from
the start, with the passage of the Rowlatt Act, which
Gandhi called "a farce of legal formality."

This was the turning-point in Gandhi's life as a politi-

cal force in India and the world. He had never taken any
direct part in politics. His work in South Africa and in
India, though political in results and implications, had all
been for the welfare of the people—social and reform
work, and in his own mind pre-eminently religious. Now
he faced a political action of great importance, from which
he did not flinch. It seemed to him that the time might
have come for an application, in India itself and on a
large scale, of the principles of *satyagraha*. He traveled
through India trying to prepare the ground for such a
movement. It was difficult to explain, as it always will be
—it seems to demand too much saintly sacrifice from
ordinary human beings—but he tried, nevertheless. He
was handicapped by his physical feebleness, found the
travel fatiguing, and was obliged to have his speeches
read for him by others. Yet he covered a great deal of
ground and put a large part of India into the frame of
mind in which some movement of non-violent protest
might be possible.

He hoped, to the end, that the Viceroy might refuse
to sign the Rowlatt Act. He wrote to the Viceroy both
privately and publicly, appealed through the press and
in every way known to him. Nevertheless the Viceroy
signed on March 18, 1919, and the Rowlatt Act became
law.

Beyond a doubt the British had no idea what they
were getting into; but it is also certain that Gandhi,
though much more enlightened, was unaware how far
these decisions would lead. He, the humble and loyal
subject of the King-Emperor, was to become a rebel. In
a sense he was a rebel from the moment the Rowlatt Act
was signed, but he did not know it for some time after-
ward. He seems to have thought of the repressive legis-

lation as, most of all, a breach of faith and a betrayal of confidence. All the kind words said to India during the war had been meaningless, for they led to this. He was not ready to renounce his allegiance to the British Raj, but he was approaching that culmination with a speed he could not have believed possible only a short time before. The place to which he had now come was not, in fact, a position in which anybody could long remain: he would have to go forward or go back. All through 1919, it seems, this necessity was obscured by day-to-day work and by the obstinacy of hope. Continued British stupidity, the massacre at Amritsar, and a mounting sense of historical destiny throughout India were to change all this within a year or two, until there was nothing left but struggle.

CHAPTER FIVE

INTO REBELLION

WHEN the Rowlatt Act became law, Gandhi was in Madras, staying in the house of C. Rajagopalachari, one of the stoutest of his lieutenants in the decades about to begin. (Rajagopalachari was known in later years as Rajaji, but for a great part of the Indian epic the news-papers called him simply "C.R.") On the morning after the signature of the act of repression Gandhi said to C.R.: "Last night in a dream the idea came to me that we should ask the whole country to observe a general *hartal*." After-wards he explained that the idea came in a state of half-dream, something between sleeping and waking.

Hartal is a day of abstention from economic activity, a day of mourning, of prayer and contemplation, some-times also of fasting. Under Gandhi's interpretation it was to be a day of fasting and prayer. (Curiously enough, the American Revolution began in much the same way: the "day of fasting and prayer" which Thomas Jefferson and his friends proclaimed for Virginia on June 1, 1774.) It was Gandhi's belief that by this means large parts of the population might be spiritually prepared for the greater efforts he intended to demand of them in the *satyagraha* campaign that he intended to undertake later. It does not seem to have weighed too much with him that the economic warning given to the British Raj would be ominous in the extreme: he did not consider this in particular because he did not expect the response to his appeal to be general. He thought Madras and Bombay,

Bihar and Sind might answer his call, and if they did, this in itself would be enough.

At first he decided upon March 30 as the day of *hartal*, and then, reflecting on the shortness of time given for orderly preparation, he changed the date to April 6.

The results were astonishing to everybody, including Gandhi. The whole of India, with few exceptions of importance, observed the day. Nobody in the great cities went to work, the banks could not operate, the ships were neither loaded nor unloaded, public transportation and even the post office were paralyzed. The complete cessation of activity proved to everybody, including the bewildered British authorities, that a new force was abroad in the land. Even though they put it all down to "sedition," and tried to treat it as such, they must have realized that it was sedition of a sort unknown before.

The *hartal* idea brought millions into the streets of India's towns and cities. Gandhi was himself in Bombay on that day (April 6) and he, with Mrs. Sarojini Naidu, spoke in a mosque. Together they sold copies of two books forbidden by the government: Gandhi's *Hind Swaraj* and his translation of Ruskin's *Unto This Last*. The government wisely decided not to arrest anybody for this, the books being "mere reprints" and therefore not the same as the books that had been proscribed. Thousands of volunteers sold copies of the books on that day and were equally unmolested.

The excitement engendered by Gandhi's appeal for *hartal* went far beyond what he had intended, and it did not stop on April 6 as he had asked. India was in turmoil. It was inevitable that heads would be broken, lives lost. The gentle Mahatma had asked too much, expected too much. Gandhi himself, in the midst of the excitement, tried to continue his journey on to Delhi and the Punjab, but was arrested on the train and turned back to Bombay. The news of his arrest, running through India like wild-fire, caused huge crowds to collect in various cities. In Bombay itself an immense mob gathered and was charged by the mounted police, with many casualties. In Ahmeda-bad, where the mill-hands were Gandhi's special chil-dren, the news of his arrest aroused a furious mob to violence, and one policeman was killed. This disturbed Gandhi more than the similar news from elsewhere, be-cause he thought the Ahmedabad workers had really understood *satyagraha*. "A rapier run through my body could scarcely have pained me more," he said.

At various times and places during these days he warned his excited followers that he would have to aban-don *satyagraha*, or even undertake a *satyagraha* of his own against his followers, if they did not carry out the principles of truth and non-violence. They had injured "some English gentlemen," and the Mahatma declared that the English were his brethren. "We have burned down buildings, forcibly captured weapons, extorted money, stopped trains, cut off telegraph wires, killed in-nocent people and plundered shops and private houses," he declared in his speech at Ahmedabad.

As a result of all this he decided that the time for *satyagraha* had not come, and he called off the move-ment. In atonement for what had happened he would fast and pray for three days, and he asked those who agreed with him to do the same thing for one day. His principles had not been understood and he would not go on until they were sufficiently understood to make the *satyagraha* pure—a sacrifice, not a violence.

No act of his life was more bewildering to the masses

in India than Gandhi's abandonment of the *satyagraha*
movement at this moment. It took a long time for Indians
in general, Hindus as well as Moslems, to understand
that the frail little man meant simply what he said, that
he had a will of iron, and that no power on earth could
induce him to pursue an action if he felt that it violated
his principles.

The Amritsar massacre took place on April 13, and
the Mahatma's abandonment of *satyagraha*, though promised in several preceding speeches, took place on April
18. The massacre coincided with his first announcement
that he intended to fast and pray. A gruesome series of
events did, in fact, follow the storm that had been summoned up by the Mahatma's dream in Madras.

The Mahatma's grief and sorrow may be imagined.
He had undertaken, in high hope, a movement that he
thought might lead to such sacrificial deeds on the part
of the Indian people that the British government would
be moved to rescind oppressive legislation and perhaps
even consider other grievances. Instead of this, his own
people had gone wild and much destruction and violence
had ensued. He had not been understood in spite of all
his patient explaining. In Bombay, instead of offering
themselves for arrest as he had asked, a great Indian
crowd surrounded the jail and clamored for the release
of fifty common criminals—precisely the opposite, as he
told them, of what he had asked.

Then, of course, the horrors of Amritsar came to add
their weight to his woe. Worst of all, he could not stir
from his *ashram*. The government of India was thoroughly aware that the great tempest now sweeping India
had come into being because of the Mahatma's request.
They therefore restricted his movements on the ground

that wherever he went he would constitute a danger to the peace. This, too, must have chafed and oppressed him— that he, whose life was given to peace, should be classi- fied as an enemy to the public order and an advocate or instigator of violence.

He wanted, above all, to go to Amritsar. But it was October of that year (1919) before he was allowed to go.

2

Amritsar, capital of the Punjab and holy city to the Sikhs, was the scene of the events of April 13, 1919, which have never been forgotten in India. In that crowded city an unprecedented show of friendship be- tween Hindu and Moslem had taken place during the *hartal* of March 30 (the original one) and the second *hartal* of April 6. However, in fear of the great crowds that had assembled, the government (of the Punjab) ordered the deportation of the two local Congress leaders, one Hindu and one Moslem, thus bringing on what they wished to avoid. The furious crowds ran amok; three English bankers were killed; others were assaulted. Briga- dier-General Reginald E. H. Dyer was ordered to Amrit- sar on April 11, and as the first act of his command (April 12) prohibited public meetings. The proclama- tion was read to the people at various points of the city, but it has never been established that its provisions were known everywhere. In any case, a public meeting took place at half past four on the afternoon of the 13th in the Jallianwalla Bagh, an open space in the middle of the city.

The Jallianwalla Bagh, in spite of its name (*bagh* is garden), has nothing of the garden about it. It is an

open space surrounded by buildings, and was then more
or less waste land with debris of one sort or another on it.
The crowd, estimated by the British official report at
somewhere between ten and twenty thousand, filled all
the space at one end and the middle. General Dyer entered on the raised ground at the opposite end with
twenty-five Gurkhas and twenty-five Baluchis, all armed
with rifles, putting one detachment on each side of him,
and then, without giving any warning or ordering the
crowd to disperse, simply opened fire and kept on firing
for ten minutes. As the exits from the Jallianwalla Bagh
are few and very narrow, it was impossible for the crowd
to get away in time. By the official British count, 379
were killed and 1,137 wounded. As the troops fired
1,650 rounds, this means that almost every bullet hit a
man.

Dyer further ordered that all Indians passing through
a certain street, where the English headmistress of a school
had been beaten by the mob on April 10, must crawl
on all fours. This applied to Indian families who had no
other means of reaching their homes. Any Indian in a
vehicle had to dismount and crawl; any Indian with a
parasol had to furl it and crawl; any Indian was ordered
to salute or salaam any English officer in these districts.
A whipping-post was installed at the spot where the
schoolmistress had been beaten, and this was used for
flogging such Indians as disobeyed any of these orders.

General Dyer always defended these well-nigh incredible actions and orders on the ground that he wished
to "make a wide impression" and a "moral effect," so as
to discourage rebellion. The official British report says:
"We have no doubt that he succeeded in creating a very
wide impression and a great moral effect, but of a char-

acter quite opposite from the one he intended." Dyer
was asked for his resignation and retired to England. Indignation in England was at a high pitch, almost as high
as in India, but without the corrosive, festering effects
of a profound national humiliation. The government in
London (Edwin Montagu being Secretary of State for
India at the time) repudiated "emphatically" the doctrine upon which Dyer based his action, and declared
that the order for Indians to crawl "offended against
every canon of civilized government."

When the whole story of the Indian national movement is viewed from the vantage point of time, it may
be seen that the massacre at Amritsar was a tragic but
decisive event. It convinced many Indians of good will
that there was no hope in British government. It pushed
Mahatma Gandhi, in his great grief, much farther into
politics (and much sooner) than he might otherwise have
gone. And truthfully, too, it inflicted many Englishmen
of good will with a sense of guilt, a desire to atone for
the outrage and to do better by India in the future. Edwin
Montagu and Lord Chelmsford (the Viceroy) were such
men, and the Montagu-Chelmsford Reforms, giving India a constitution and a share in government, were proposed in that same year, 1919.

But the bitterness of Amritsar was responsible for
many of India's vicissitudes in the next twenty years—
for the widespread belief that the British were never to
be trusted; for the difficulties of any negotiation; for sporadic acts of violence; for a growth of downright enmity,
of inimical feelings, on both sides. Seldom can one officer
of fairly modest rank have produced such a tangle of historical results from one decision. General Dyer was a
product of his particular class and climate (born in India,

educated in an Irish Tory school, and commissioned in
the army at nineteen), but this fact in itself pointed up
every evil of the regime, which Indians of every class
were now beginning to detest.

3

Mahatma Gandhi was unable to get to Amritsar all
summer long. Finally Lord Chelmsford telegraphed him
that he was free to go "any time after October 17th."
(We may speculate that the reforms had already been
decided upon in London and that this was a sign of the
coming attempt at conciliation.) Wherever he went, he
was received by those delirious crowds who then and
thereafter were never to leave him. The demonstrations
in Lahore, a city of many Moslems, were particularly
striking. In Amritsar he settled down to make his own inquiry into the massacre of Jallianwalla Bagh. Motilal
Nehru, father of Jawaharlal, who was not only a Congress
leader of great prestige but a first-class lawyer, worked
with Gandhi on this report, as did a number of other men
of repute in the Congress, but the actual drafting was
left to the Mahatma.

Gandhi had never been to the Punjab before, and
seems not to have realized how powerful a symbol he had
become, there as elsewhere in India. He actually said to
the police in Bombay, when they first prevented him
from going to the Punjab in April: "Nobody knows me
there." The excitement surrounding his visit must have
convinced him to the contrary. Thousands of Punjabis
filed before him to tell their stories, and he listened as
patiently as always, though he rejected anything he
thought exaggerated or unproved. The official British

report had been prepared on much less evidence than
this unofficial one of Gandhi's, because the British inquiry had been boycotted by most of the Indians who
could have testified. Whether Gandhi's inquiry or the
official one corresponds more closely to the facts can
hardly be determined now; they differed chiefly in the
numbers given for dead and wounded. But the principal
result of the inquiry, in Gandhi's life, was that it en-
twined him more closely into political life than before;
having made this inquiry, he could not refuse to take
part in the annual meeting of the Congress that year (in
Amritsar) or in the Hindu-Moslem conversations on the
Caliphate. The process that had begun with his dream
in Madras was quite relentlessly leading him into the
central position in Indian and empire politics, whether
he desired it or not.

The progression was accelerated by the question of
the Caliphate of Islam, considered vital by the Mohammedans of India. Gandhi had been by instinct, nature,
and deliberate intention a friend of the Moslems all his
life. He once said in South Africa, long before he returned to India, that the final test of his *satyagraha* would
come on Hindu-Moslem unity. Now an opportunity was
offered to make that unity real, and he could not refuse
it. He left Amritsar for Delhi in November 1919 for the
Moslem Conference, to which he had been officially invited. The Moslems were so eager for his support that
they offered to place cow-protection on the agenda of
their conference: Gandhi felt the artificiality of the proposal, and refused. If Moslems wished to respect Hindu
susceptibilities by ceasing the slaughter of cows, they
could do so, and it had nothing to do with the Caliphate.

If Hindus wished to support Moslem desires for the Caliphate of Islam they should do so without attempting to
make a bargain on cow-protection.

Gandhi was on the platform at this fateful Moslem conference, listening to all the debate. The Moslems of India had already passed resolutions condemning the British for being too severe with Turkey; the time had now
come to think of some method of making their desires
felt. All expected that the final peace terms dictated to
Turkey would truncate that old Moslem state and destroy the Caliphate of Islam, the center of the Moslem
world.

Gandhi's contribution, when it came his time to speak,
was the single momentous word "non-cooperation." He
could not very well propose to Mohammedans the idea
of *satyagraha*, which was too far-reaching, too profound,
and too difficult to understand. *Satyagraha* was not in the
Moslem tradition or character; indeed, it was supernally
difficult for most Hindus. The word itself was Sanskrit
and therefore not suited to the English-speaking Moslems
of this conference. Gandhi, after days of reflection, decided upon "non-cooperation" as the suitable English
word.

A boycott of English textiles, as the Moslems had
proposed, was not in itself a sufficient action. What was
needed, Gandhi told them, was a firm non-cooperation
in all other fields: a refusal of British employment, British honors, British schools or courts. With the entire ma-
chinery of British government in India—up to, as was
later included, the non-payment of taxes—the Moslems
should undertake non-cooperation at the risk of much
personal sacrifice and loss. So grave a step should not be
taken, however, unless the British terms of peace with

Turkey were fully known; if they were as severe as expected, non-cooperation was the right response.

The word and the idea dominated Indian public life
for years afterwards. And yet in a new test that came
within a month, Gandhi was in favor of co-operation
with the British.

This was the Montagu-Chelmsford Reforms, as they
were called from the names of their authors: a first step
toward constitutional government in India. The Reforms
were announced on the day before the Indian National
Congress held its annual meeting at Amritsar. The constitutional system devised was unsatisfactory to all other
Indians, Gandhi said, "and was not wholly satisfactory
even to me," but he thought it wiser to accept the proposals in good faith and try them out as a beginning.

By this time Gandhi's power over the masses in India
was already so great that the lawyers and pundits of the
National Congress could not go on without him. When
he discovered that the Congress as a whole disagreed
with him, and did not wish to accept the Montagu-
Chelmsford Reforms, he tried to retire to his *ashram*
rather than argue it out. They would not let him go
away—any decision taken in his absence would have
been almost meaningless to the people of India, because
the mere fact of his absence would have indicated disapproval. Thus, again, circumstance maneuvered the drama
in such a way that Gandhi's words and moves, or even
his silences, exercised a fateful spell over political evolution. Under these circumstances he stayed in the Congress, and although he disliked having to overcome some
of its veteran leaders who disagreed with him, he stated
his views and they prevailed. The Congress passed a
resolution commending the Reforms and thanking Ed-

win Montagu, but asking for the recall of Lord Chelmsford for mismanagement. (The Viceroy had defended Dyer after the Amritsar massacre.) The other resolutions passed also followed the general recommendations of Gandhi, who from this time forward was the unquestioned spirit of the Indian National Congress, impossible to disregard even when his wishes were most tentatively expressed and even when they ran counter to the wishes of the impatient youth of the country.

Gandhi himself, however, rapidly lost faith in the good intentions of the British. Aside from Edwin Montagu, nobody in the government in London seemed to realize what the abolition of the Caliphate meant to the Moslems of India. A ruthless peace treaty was dictated to Turkey. The Hindus of India at the same time were flouted by the fact that General Dyer's pension (paid by India) was continued after his retirement to England, and by the fact that a large purse was collected there as a gift to him in sympathy after the Amritsar massacre. These and many other episodes—the continued enforcement of the Rowlatt Act being one—finally drove Gandhi into the acceptance (April 1920) of the presidency of the Home Rule League. This was a symbolic deed, placing him on record as an opponent of the existing government, though not yet as an outright rebel. It was much farther than he had ever gone before. The organ of political action continued to be the Indian National Congress, of which the Home Rulers were also members, but Gandhi's adherence to home rule gave the idea a powerful impetus.

The time for active non-cooperation had now come. Gandhi's advice impelled the Khilafat (Caliphate) movement to adopt it as a policy, and his own word was

enough to ensure Hindu support. He wrote to the Viceroy, as was his custom, giving due and courteous notice
that he had advised the Moslems and Hindus "to with-
draw their support from Your Excellency's government."
The Viceroy said that non-cooperation was "the most
foolish of all foolish schemes."

Gandhi asked for a day of fasting and prayer throughout India on July 31. Non-cooperation would begin on
August 1.

It was very far from being a "foolish scheme" as it
worked out. Hindu and Moslem committees, working
together, scoured the country and induced millions to
give up their British clothing and even jobs. Gandhi himself was incessantly moving about India, immune to fa-
tigue, preaching his home-rule gospel in the Hindi word
swaraj (self-rule). He had completely dominated the
special Congress held in early September 1920, just
after the beginning of non-cooperation. That Congress
adopted non-cooperation, and it was confirmed by the
regular annual meeting at Nagpur in December. At Nagpur, Gandhi produced a constitution for the Congress
(which had had none before): it created the system of
village, district, and city units, the executive All-India
Congress Committee of 350, and a Working Committee of fifteen, the system under which the organization
has endured. Thus the body of upper middle-class lawyers, bankers, and pundits, brought into being originally by the British, became a mass organization with its
roots deep in Indian life.

Gandhi's tours during late 1920 and the greater part
of 1921 took him everywhere in the country that could
be reached by railroad, and into many districts where
the railroad did not go. It was his habit to ask for the

sacrifice of foreign clothing, and the great bonfires that
soon burned all over India were actually started by him.
Sometimes men stripped themselves naked and put all
their clothes on the great central heap. When he had finished speaking, the Mahatma himself applied the match
to the fire. The example was followed all over India,
and women of the upper classes vied with one another
in sacrificing textiles bought from England. Men and
women were taking to the spinning-wheel, which now
began to be produced in quantity, and it was part of the
Mahatma's plea that they should all get into homespun
as soon as possible.

At that time he wore homespun, but the garments
themselves were conventional enough: a white cap
(known thereafter as the "Gandhi cap"), a dhoti, or
loosely draped trousers, and a sleeveless vest. It was not
until September 1921 that he took the final step and
adopted the dress of the poorest of the poor—a loincloth
and, in cold weather, a homespun shawl.

During this period money was collected on a very
great scale. A spirit of sacrifice swept over India, as it
did periodically thereafter during the Mahatma's active
campaigns. This was perhaps the highest, as it was the
first, of these general passionate assertions of belief in the
Mahatma's way to freedom. It is remarkable indeed that
in the midst of all this excitement, with great crowds almost constant in the cities and towns, violence did not
occur anywhere for many months.

Gandhi traveled for a large part of the time with Mohammed Ali, younger of the two brothers who were ac-
knowledged leaders of the Moslems. It was a high point,
too, of Hindu-Moslem unity. Yet in September 1921
Mohammed Ali was arrested and Gandhi was not,

though they were walking together to a meeting at the time. The arrest was made because Mohammed Ali had asked Moslems not to join the British army; his elder brother went to jail for the same offense soon afterwards. Gandhi, in great distress at the loss of his Moslem friend and fellow worker, asked the Congress Working Committee (October 5) to pass a resolution declaring it the duty of every Indian soldier or civilian to quit the government service—thus sharing whatever guilt the Ali brothers had incurred.

It was just at this point that Gandhi went to the final extreme in simplicity of clothing and adopted the loincloth as being the garment of the poor.

The government of India may or may not have been responsible for the visit of the Prince of Wales at the end of the year: it was probably a miscalculation on the part of the London government, influenced by the Prince's immense popularity at that time in Europe and America. Perhaps it was thought that he could calm the tempest in India. Instead of doing so, he added to it. His parades through empty streets in some cities and through demonstrations of hostility in others should have been a serious warning. Unfortunately, the royal visit aroused even more emotional tensions among the Indians themselves, and violence broke out. In Bombay the nationalists made an attack on those Indians who had, in spite of the boycott, gone out to welcome the Prince, and the ensuing riots were a terrible additional grief to the Mahatma. He undertook to fast as a prayer for peace until the violence should cease, and took no food for five days.

It is often asked, even now, why the British authorities refrained from arresting Gandhi in 1921, at a time when others were being arrested on a very large scale for

doing what he asked them to do. By the end of the year
some twenty thousand Indians were in jail for obeying
Gandhi's wishes (sedition, it was called), and over the
turn of the year ten thousand more joined them.

It is easy to say, and often has been said, that the government was fearful of the results that might ensue, in a
climate so agitated, if the Mahatma was sent to prison.
That fear no doubt played some part. But it is known
now that the new Viceroy, Lord Reading, was almost
alone responsible for the immunity the Mahatma enjoyed (or, in fact, did not enjoy—it worried him a good
deal). Lord Reading was a man of very exceptional
quality indeed, and had risen to his eminence by his own
efforts. (He started life as a messenger boy on a ship,
and was afterwards a fruit merchant before he studied the
law.) On his arrival in India, in April of this year, 1921,
he had wanted to talk to Gandhi and had proceeded to
do so at great length, though they were both criticized by
their own friends for consenting to the interviews at such
a moment. The details were all published by Reading's
son in a biography that appeared long afterwards
(1945), complete with the Viceroy's own letters home
on the subject.

In these very curious conversations, six in number,
Gandhi attempted to inculcate his ideas of truth, non-
violence, and love on the worldly-wise Viceroy. Reading obviously was rather startled at first, as he had no
doubt been coached by the British "experts" on India to
expect a crafty and guileful Babu. He was quick to rec-
ognize the sincerity, courtesy, and, as he says, "distinction" of his visitor, and declared at once that the moral
and religious views of Gandhi were "on a remarkably
high altitude." He could not see, however, how the Ma-

hatma was to apply them in practical politics. The Mahatma explained, as he always did, that the first task for Indians was self-purification by means of non-violence, truth, and love, and that in this process the English rule ("white supremacy") would cease naturally as a result. (I myself do not think the Mahatma ever used an expression like "white supremacy," which sounds to me like Reading's own paraphrase.)

Lord Reading may have been puzzled: so it seems. But he was also tremendously impressed. It is quite possible that he felt in Gandhi's presence, as others felt before and after, a sort of unearthly purity before which all ordinary considerations became vulgar and insignificant. Whether this was true or not, the fact is that the Viceroy remained for many months unwilling to order Gandhi's arrest, sometimes standing alone against it while the government in London and the governors of the Indian provinces were all demanding it.

The British were not alone in being puzzled by the Mahatma's course during 1921 and early 1922. Many Indians, impatient and angry, wanted to begin an armed rebellion. They were restrained by the knowledge that Gandhi would never approve of it, and that without his approval the masses would not move. Thus both the Indian nationalists and the British faced a situation so new that it was impossible for either of them to evaluate it properly and difficult for them both to take any decision.

The arrests continued until practically all Indian leaders except Gandhi were in prison. In the annual Congress meeting at the end of 1921 there was little to do except what the Congress did do: elect Gandhi as the "sole executive authority."

He was now in complete control of the situation. His

slightest word was law for millions. India, and a very large part of the world besides, waited anxiously for what he would do next. The more impatient nationalists were urging him to go beyond non-cooperation into outright civil disobedience and to do this on the largest possible scale immediately, since the situation was obviously (they thought) of a revolutionary nature and temperature. Nobody dared to advocate violence in his presence (and by this time very few Indians dared to appear before him in European clothing). But civil disobedience on a vast scale, involving over three hundred million people, might very well lead to violence, and no doubt the advocates of violence (Bengali and others) counted upon that.

However, out of his endless self-communing and meditation, the Mahatma brought forth a new idea. He would try a campaign of civil disobedience, under his own direction, in one circumscribed district, where his own presence and influence might keep the people within the limits of his principles. He did not hope for pure *satyagraha*, actual pure sacrifice, but for a campaign of straight, non-violent civil disobedience in which no Indian would in any way assist the British government or public services to carry out their functions.

He chose the small district of Bardoli, in the Bombay Presidency, for this experiment. It had a population of eighty-seven thousand, mostly in small villages, where the danger of violence was less than in cities. Even in a small district, however, the total paralysis of all British authority would be a solemn warning to the government. Gandhi hoped that the warning might be heeded and that no more extreme measures would become necessary. He was by nature both cautious and optimistic, and the Bardoli experiment, so modest in comparison with the schemes of others, corresponded to his sense of right.

He therefore wrote to Lord Reading on February 1, 1922, and courteously informed him of the decision he had taken.

The All-India Congress Committee had actually gone on record the preceding November in favor of a civil-disobedience campaign for the entire country, and Gandhi, much disquieted, had exacted from them a promise to do nothing without his consent. Under the circumstances the greatest force for the preservation of order in India was not the British government, army, or police, but the fragile little man of Sabarmati.

He went to Bardoli and prepared to set about his task. As usual, he was eager for the people to understand that success in the movement could be achieved only if no violence was offered, and that no resistance should be made to any police action. He emphasized, as always, the importance of prayer and a reliance upon religious faith in any pure action. While he was thus busied, the news reached him (February 8) of a dreadful atrocity.

It occurred at Chauri Chaura in the United Provinces. By Gandhi's own account, written in his weekly paper *Young India* on February 16, a legal procession had taken place there without police interference, but after it was over some stragglers were molested by the constables. The stragglers called for help. In Gandhi's words: "The mob returned. The constables opened fire. The little ammunition they had was exhausted and they retired to the Thana for safety. The mob, my informant tells me, therefore set fire to the Thana. The self-imprisoned constables had to come out for dear life and as they did so they were hacked to pieces and the mangled remains were thrown into the raging flames."

This horror so depressed the Mahatma that again, as in 1919, he felt compelled to cancel the entire campaign of civil disobedience, not only in the Bardoli district, but everywhere in India. In penitence for the crime committed at Chauri Chaura he fasted for five days while both India and Great Britain looked on in amazement. It seemed hardly possible, at that time, that a man could go so far toward revolution—bloodless and peaceful, but still revolution—and then call it off with a prayer. However, it was Gandhi's way, and the masses did as he said, not as any other might tell them. To the Indians who protested, the Mahatma said patiently: "The drastic reversal of practically the whole of the aggressive program may be politically unsound and unwise, but there is no doubt that it is religiously sound."

Lord Reading, who had held off for so long against those in London and India who wanted Gandhi arrested, now decided, rather mysteriously, to give the order. In his letters to his son he had said that he was waiting for an "overt act," his democratic feelings being all against arresting anybody for words alone. The only "overt act" Gandhi committed in February was one of peace, renunciation, and penitence for the Chauri Chaura atrocity, and yet the governors of the great provinces (Lloyd, Willingdon, and Ronaldshay) still wanted him arrested. The Viceroy issued the order on March 1, 1922, and it was executed on March 10 at half past ten at night.

The Mahatma had anticipated his own arrest for a long time and had published an appeal, one day before the arrest took place, asking the people to be calm if the event occurred. It is quite probable that he had been disappointed at his prolonged exemption from the punishment his whole system courted. The British—misunderstanding as usual—thought that his imprisonment "like an ordinary mortal" was a "blow to his prestige," remaining unaware, even at this late date, that such imprisonment was a calculated part of the *satyagraha* and that Gandhi's system would not have been complete without it. They also seem not to have realized (at least the Viceroy did not) that India's quiet and good order were in obedience to the Mahatma's wishes rather than to the power of the British Raj.

The trial took place in Ahmedabad on March 18, 1922. Gandhi and the printer of his magazine, Mr. S. G. Banker, were charged with writing and publishing three seditious articles in *Young India*. They were, indeed, seditious: the first of them declares it in so many words ("sedition has become the creed of the Congress"). It also declares it a sin for any soldier or civilian to serve the government. The second article proclaims rebellion and asks the government to understand that this is war. The third article asserts that the war will go on to the end, no matter how long it may take.

The first of these articles, which in effect invited arrest, had appeared seven months before. It must have been puzzling to many then, as it still is to us, why the arrest had not been made when the article first came out. One might be tempted to think that the British held off precisely because Gandhi wanted to be arrested, but on the contrary they do not seem to have understood that this was his wish. The stupidity of even such a very clever man as Lord Reading is startling in retrospect, but Gandhi's methods were new then and difficult for his contemporaries to comprehend.

A great show of military force was made at Ahmedabad during the trial. It was, of course, unnecessary, as the people there and throughout India understood the Mahatma's wishes and obeyed them. The attention of the whole country (and, for the first time, of the entire world) centered upon Gandhi that day. He did not defend himself against the charges—indeed, he stated that he was more seditious, and had been more seditious for a longer time, than the government's case charged. He asked the judge, if he believed in this law and this government, to impose the highest penalty that could be inflicted.

The Mahatma's statement, outlining his transformation from a loyal subject of the Raj into a rebel against it, had tremendous effect at the time. His behavior still had, in 1922, the element of surprise—people in general were not used to him, and they seem to have thought he would defend himself somehow, or at least ask for mercy. We who follow afterwards can see that such would never be his way, that he would be compelled by his entire inner logic to demand the maximum punishment.

The judge, Mr. C. N. Broomfield, was obviously embarrassed, regretful. His was no easy task. "It will be impossible to ignore the fact that you are in a different category from any person I have ever tried or am likely to have to try," he said. He went on to say that Gandhi was a "great patriot and a great leader" in the eyes of millions. "Even those who differ from you in politics look upon you as a man of high ideals and of noble and even saintly life."

The sentence imposed was six years of simple imprisonment. "If the course of events in India should make it possible for the government to reduce the period and release you," said the judge, "no one will be better pleased than I."

Gandhi stated that this was as mild a sentence as could have been imposed by any judge; one can tell by his words that he was feeling rather sorry for Mr. Broomfield. He also remarked upon the great courtesy with which he had been treated in the proceedings. He was led away between kneeling and weeping spectators.

It is worth pointing out once again that imprisonment was not only welcome to Gandhi, but absolutely essential. His system depended upon it. Moreover, he never asked others to do anything he was not willing to do himself: it had been a fundamental rule for many years, and it applied to imprisonment just as it did to digging latrines or washing dirty clothes. It was so much a cardinal point in his eyes that he never tired of repeating it. Consequently, for him to remain any longer out of jail when so many thousands of his followers were locked up would have violated his sense of justice and caused him great grief. Quite possibly the cleverest thing the British could have done would have been never to arrest him at all: it is possible, though not likely, that he would have abandoned public life if he had been immune to punishment while others suffered. One cannot tell at this distance. In any case, the British were not clever, so (as the Mahatma would say) "the contingency did not arise."

4

Gandhi was quite happy in Yeravda Jail, where he was lodged in solitary confinement from March 20, 1922, to January 12, 1924. He said himself, in one of his letters from jail, that he was "happy as a bird." His life outside of prison was so totally public at all times, and was lived in proximity to so many persons, that incarceration had a genuine appeal to the solitary and contemplative elements of his nature. The British were extremely courteous to him, and when they realized that he had taken a vow to spin every day, they broke their own rules and allowed a spinning-wheel to be brought into the cell. This was, however, the only special privilege he was willing to accept. He refused to be transferred to a special section of the jail and also wrote to the governor of the prison saying he wanted no dietary privileges if other prisoners did not have them.

Four hours of each day he spent at the spinning-wheel—a source of immense happiness to him. In life outside of prison he had never been able to get in more than an hour's spinning a day. The wheel no doubt had a fundamental mystic significance, as it does throughout the Indic and Buddhist world, but for Gandhi it had also an almost immeasurable practical importance for "the economic salvation of impoverished India." For these and other reasons, a complex of reasons, he grew steadily more devoted to spinning. He learned carding and weaving (had just learned carding when he went to prison), but his first and last love was the wheel.

The rest of his long day (four in the morning to eight at night) was given to books, correspondence, and meditation. The *Gita* took a good part of his time, as always, but he also read the *Koran* and some Christian literature. This happy existence was brought to an end by a sudden appendicitis.

The dilemma of the British was painful. They could not permit him to die in jail, but neither could they risk an unsuccessful operation. They transferred him in haste to the Sassoon Hospital in Poona, where the Mahatma signed a declaration, in the presence of two Indian friends summoned for the purpose, saying that he had consented to the operation for appendicitis, and that, whatever happened to him, the people of India should not make it a pretext for agitation against the government. This precaution was highly necessary, for at the mere rumor of his illness excitement began to rise all over the country.

The operation, by a colonel of the British Medical Corps, was successful, though performed under difficulties (the electricity went off and the job was done by the light of a hurricane lantern). The government of India (or perhaps that in London) decided that under the circumstances Gandhi had been in prison long enough, and on February 5 he was released. In the midst of a great outburst of national rejoicing, he went to Juhu Beach, near Bombay, to spend his convalescence in the house of a well-to-do friend.

Gandhi's term in prison (almost two years) had undone much of his most cherished work. The Congress party had passed into the hands of the activists, C. R. Das and Motilal Nehru, who wished to participate in provincial councils and in general in dyarchy politics; all the boycotts were dead or dying: lawyers were returning to their practice and students to their colleges; non-cooperation had ceased and there had been no civil disobedience since Gandhi had himself canceled it. But worst, much the worst of all in Gandhi's eyes, Hindu-Moslem unity had been shattered, and there had been communal riots, violence, and murder in a number of places.

Under these circumstances Gandhi, who did not want to split the nationalists into factions, decided to leave pol-

itics to others and devote himself to what he called "constructive work." He adhered to this line for several years,
but in point of fact everything he said or did had some influence on politics because he was the focus of attention
for all India and the masses would have no other guru.
His "constructive work" itself had vast political effects—
the spinning-wheel, for instance, and his work for the untouchables. He was not now, and never had been, anti-
British; he held that the key to *Swaraj* (self-rule) for India was not in British, but in Indian hands. India would
be free when it was purified, and not before.

In this task of "purifying India" it was obvious that
the first thing must be a restoration of friendliness between Hindus and Moslems. As soon as his strength was
partially restored, Gandhi resumed the editorship of his
weekly paper, *Young India* (he called it his "viewspa-
per"), and of the Gujarati monthly *Navajivan*. Both had
large circulations, but *Young India* during these years
was eagerly read throughout the country, as it was in
English, which was, and is, the one language common
to all regions. In *Young India* Gandhi returned again and
again to the subject of Hindu-Moslem relations, which
were not only bad, but actually were deteriorating. He
had many words of stern common sense to say about the
communal clashes.

In the summer of 1924 things went from bad to
worse between the two communities. Not only did violence happen in crowded cities where mobs got out of
hand, but actually many Indians, including members of
the Congress Working Committee, believed in violence
as a method or means. When Ghandi went to a meeting
of the Working Committee that June and was made to
understand that a considerable number of his own asso-

ciates did not believe in his non-violence, he wept publicly. They had followed his non-violent campaign of two years before because it seemed to be getting results, not because they believed in it as a principle. This was a great grief to him.

On September 18, 1924, therefore, he had recourse to his supreme remedy and declared a fast of twenty-one days devoted to the prayer for peace between Hindu and Moslem.

His physical condition made this an extremely temerarious undertaking, and yet, upon the evidence, it seems clear that nothing else could have brought peace to India. The Mahatma had been writing and speaking on the subject ever since his release from prison, and the situation had grown steadily worse. He felt then, as he was to feel so often afterwards, that people no longer listened to him: they could come out by the million to see him, to kneel beside his train as it passed them, even to touch the dust that his feet had trodden, but they would not really listen to what he had to say. The "craze for darshan," as he called it—the desire of the masses to receive the mystical blessing that is supposed to come from the sight of a saint or even of a great leader of men—got in the way of his work. And it was indeed true that many gazed upon the Mahatma with reverence and with love, but listened to not a word he was saying: I saw this with my own eyes. In earlier days it was not possible for most of them to listen, anyhow, as his voice was ever feeble and there were no microphones: how could a crowd of twenty-five thousand people do anything but catch a glimpse of him? As for reading, it was truer then than now that most Indians were illiterate.

In announcing the great fast of 1924 Gandhiji referred sadly to this state of affairs. "Nothing, evidently," he said, "which I say or write can bring the two communities together. I am therefore imposing on myself a twenty-one-day fast from today and ending Wednesday October 6th. I reserve the liberty to drink water with or without salt. It is both a penance and a prayer. . . . I respectfully invite the heads of all communities, including Englishmen, to meet and end this quarrel which is a disgrace to religion and to humanity. It seems as if God has been dethroned. Let us reinstate Him in our hearts."

The sources of Gandhi's power over the masses of Indians, and to a lesser degree over all his contemporaries, were numerous and complex, but high among them must be named the instinct for symbolic action. Certain of his most characteristic acts (such as this fast, and later the Salt March) carried the stamp of a peculiar genius, one that knew how to dramatize the truth. There was no theater in this twenty-one-day fast: it was grim torture part of the time and profoundly serious all of the time. Yet it conveyed to the most ignorant villager the truth of a great sacrifice for peace. Because it was true and felt by everybody to be true, its effect was immediate and magical. Long before the fast was over, Hindus and Moslems, with prayer and weeping, had pledged themselves by the millions to keep the peace.

Mohammed Ali, Gandhi's friend of the 1921 campaign, had a house in Delhi, and it was there, sheltered by Moslems and cared for by Moslem doctors, that the Mahatma chose to undergo his ordeal. His last food before, and his first food after, the fast would thus be given him by Moslems. (The administration of food has special significance in Hinduism, and is governed by caste regulations.) His great friend, the Christian missionary Charles Freer Andrews ("Charlie"), acted as his nurse. The prayers and hymns at the beginning and the end of the epic endeavor were Moslem, Christian, and Hindu, all three. In every respect the dramatization, if one may call it that, of the Mahatma's truth was carried out so that the whole world could see what religious unity might mean and might achieve if it could come into being for all as it did for this one.

It must be said at once, of course, that religious unity was not brought into effect on the practical stage of history by the Mahatma's great fast. The fast had tremendous immediate results, but all, unfortunately, based upon fear for Gandhi's life. By this time it had become impossible for anybody in India to imagine what life would be like without the Mahatma. (At the time of his assassination this was at the root of the semi-paralysis that seemed to have overtaken everybody one saw.) The fear of his death produced a temporary unity and millions of peace pledges, but in stony fact the enmity between Hindu and Moslem did not really diminish, and in subsequent years actually increased.

The thing in itself, however, held the imagination of the world for those three weeks, and it is still difficult for many to remember it without a stir of emotion. Nothing of the kind, no symbol of such incontrovertible purity, had been offered the world for a very long time. With considerable gaiety at times, and always in good spirits, the fragile little man affronted risks that are seldom taken either in war or for peace. He seems to have had some inner assurance that he could fast three weeks without a danger of suicide—suicide, which, as he told me himself

by implication, he had always rejected. His assurance
came from his "inner voice," which seems to have been
remarkably right on all the occasions known to us.

He ended the fast exactly as it had been planned, on
Wednesday, October 6, at midday. Before accepting a
glass of orange juice from his Moslem doctor, the Mahatma asked for a little religious ceremony. The Imam
recited the opening verses of the Koran. Charlie Andrews
sang "When I Survey the Wondrous Cross" in English.
Vinoba Bhave recited (in Sanskrit) from the Upanishads, and the favorite Vaishnava hymn was sung. Many
of the leaders of the Indian National Congress were in
the room, seated on the floor near the bed. The Mahatma spoke very briefly, in a barely audible voice, before the service, asking those present to be ready to give
their lives for brotherhood.

5

In the years preceding the great struggle that reached
its climax in the Salt March (1930), Gandhi devoted
himself almost entirely to his "constructive work," and
most of all to the spinning-wheel. His desire to revive
that instrument of salvation, as he called it, was bearing
fruit; more and more Indians were learning to spin, more
and more wheels were coming forth, more homespun was
being worn. In 1925 the All-Indian Spinners' Association was formed to press forward the work. Gandhi himself made incessant long tours throughout the country,
visiting every province and state in turn, always pursuing
his aim of the "purification of India." His teaching was
not always received by the minds of those who formed
his audiences, as we have seen, but his moral authority
was as supreme when he ignored politics as when he took

an active part. Nothing of which he really disapproved could get far in Indian political life because, no matter where he was or what he was doing, his disapproval would somehow come out and be instantly known throughout the country.

Thus he was never "out of power," even when he turned his back on political life and worked for the spinning-wheel or the villagers. He was never "out of power" and never "in power," in the Western sense: he simply *was* power, so far as India was concerned, and never to be gainsaid.

The years 1924–8 are remarkable, as Louis Fischer has pointed out in his *Life of Mahatma Gandhi*, for the fact that in all of Gandhi's voluminous speaking and writing there is little reference to the English or to British rule. He was at this period intent on "*Swaraj* from within" —that is, on preparing India, by "purification" and endless teaching, for the pure *satyagraha* that would some day be possible and would bring freedom. In this preparation the British had no part and the question of foreign rule was irrelevant: it was Indians who had to be made ready from within, Indians who must learn to be clean and truthful and to spin and weave their cloth and walk uprightly with their God. The time for the British would come later, when Indians had been made ready.

Thus he toured and worked and walked and talked. Wherever he went, there were vast crowds and his feet were often injured or scratched by the innumerable persons who attempted to touch them. In many of his meetings in behalf of homespun (*khadi*) and the wheel (*charkha*), ladies or young girls gave him their jewels, which he cheerfully accepted and put to use in the work for the spinning-wheel.

Fischer dates the "deification" of Gandhi from these years; I should have thought it started a little earlier. In any case there is no doubt that he was much plagued during the 1920's by various outbursts of excessive reverence touching on worship. He did not like it. One tribe, the Gonds, had deified him outright, to his "horror and strongest disapproval." He was represented in temples from about 1924 or 1925 on, and one southern temple is said to have been dedicated to him in the mid-1920's. His dislike for these excesses of the Indian religious instinct was strong. He realized, of course, that the Western mind could not understand such things, and undoubtedly he feared for India the ridicule of the foreigners, as well as the harm that such deification could very well do to his own work. As a Hindu he knew that there was nothing inherently improper, or contrary to the religion, in taking one man to represent an aspect of the divine principle: such has been Hindu practice since before records began, and it is the fundamental Hindu doctrine that divinity dwells in all life, immanent and transcendent. Gandhi, however, may have had too much Western thought sifted through his own consciousness to accept this, at least with regard to himself; he never really accepted even the appellation "Mahatma," much less any more extreme form of distinction.

Most of all, he seems to have been embarrassed by legend and miracle. He tried to laugh them out of existence. A man traveling on a train with him fell out, landed on his head, and came up smiling. His miraculous escape, he said, had been due to the fact that he was traveling with the Mahatma. The Mahatma said: "But in that case you wouldn't have fallen out at all." A poor man in Bengal came to him wearing a photograph of the

Mahatma on a chain around his neck; the man had been paralyzed, he said, and by endlessly repeating the name of Gandhi he had, after many years, been cured. "It was God who cured you, not Gandhi," the Mahatma said sharply, "and kindly oblige me by taking that photograph off your neck."

All these phenomena of the living legend were to be expected, above all in India, but do not seem to have been expected by the Mahatma; he was in this respect, as in so many others having to do with himself, an incurable innocent, with a naïveté seldom equaled.

When he first came out of jail, Gandhi had said that he intended to retire from the Indian National Congress and from political life. The spontaneous protest that arose from the whole country delayed him a bit; in fact, he was persuaded to accept the presidency of the Congress for 1925. He accepted it on one condition: that the Congress should take to wearing homespun, should make it an article of Congress doctrine, and should not admit any member who would not wear it. Wherever and whenever possible, every member of Congress was to spin an hour each day. The Congress—then badly split in political views—could not do without Gandhi; he as president could preserve their unity; they all accepted *khadi*, and from 1925 onward it became the official wear for all Indian nationalists.

One fast he undertook toward the end of 1925 (November) without giving a public explanation. It lasted for seven days and aroused endless speculation and bewilderment in India. Gandhi did not see why he had to explain.

"The public will have to neglect my fasts and cease to worry about them," he wrote in *Young India*. "They are part of my being. I can as well do without my eyes, for instance, as I can without fasts. What the eyes are for the outer world, fasts are for the inner." And, later on: "This fast has nothing to do with the public. It is said, I am public property. . . . So be it. But I must be taken with all my faults. I am a searcher after truth. My experiments I hold to be infinitely more important than the best-equipped Himalayan expeditions."

In 1926, when his year's presidency of the Congress was at an end, Mahatma declared a year of "political silence." It was not a silence in other respects, but he vowed to say nothing on political subjects until the year was over, and to remain in his own *ashram*, or at least in its neighborhood, all that time. ("No farther away than Ahmedabad" he would go.) There is no doubt that he needed a rest, body and soul; perhaps his body set up warning signals, or the "inner voice" admonished him. He was certainly not idle during the year, and his voluminous correspondence alone was enough to keep him busy on many subjects. *Young India* was the organ through which India heard (and promptly reprinted in all the public press) what the Mahatma was thinking.

On the sexual questions that filled *Young India* Gandhi made a long series of pertinent answers during the year. He recognized the need for birth control in India, but wanted to see it brought about by the method of self-control. He ceaselessly advocated late marriages, bland diets, vegetarianism of the strictest sort, exercise, and a reliance on prayer and work as means to controlling sexual desire. He attacked child marriage as vehemently as he did untouchability and other evils; the existence of child widows (who could not remarry under Hindu law) was a great horror to him. He gave the British figures for

1921: 329,076 widows under sixteen in India, 11,892 of them less than five years old, and 85,037 of them between five and ten. He permitted girls in his *ashram* to marry only after they had reached the age of twenty-one, and in print he advocated twenty-five as the marriage age for boys. By all these means he hoped to bring down the birth rate without having recourse to artificial contraceptives, which were repugnant to him on religious grounds.

Lord Irwin (later Lord Halifax), the new Viceroy, arrived in India on April 1, 1926. Gandhi did not mention this in *Young India*, and it was over a year and a half before the Viceroy sent for Gandhi. By this time it was October 1927 and the Mahatma had finished his "year of silence" and was again touring India. He had fallen ill and gone through a long and difficult convalescence during the greater part of 1927. Now he journeyed to Delhi to see the Viceroy and was confronted with a strange bit of paper announcing that Sir John Simon would soon arrive in India at the head of a Parliamentary commission of inquiry on Indian conditions, with the power to recommend reforms. Gandhi accepted the paper in silence and departed without comment.

The Simon Commission was doomed from the start because it contained no Indian members and was responsible only to the British Parliament. It was the creation of Lord Birkenhead, then Secretary of State for India, whose oratory had made him famous in the courts of law but was singularly unsuited to the realities he now faced. "What man in this House," Birkenhead asked in the Commons in 1929, "can say that he can see in a generation, in two generations, in a hundred years, any prospect that the people of India will be in a position to assume control of the Army, the Navy, the Civil Service,

and to have a Governor-General who will be responsible
to the Indian government and not to any authority in this
country?"

The Simon Commisson was boycotted by all responsible groups and parties in India. It arrived in Bombay
on February 2, 1928, to be greeted by crowds yelling
"Go back, Simon." It was surrounded by hostility
throughout the time of its labors, and produced a report
which, though full of facts, might as well never have
been written. As a work of reference it is still used; as a
political document it was a dead letter.

On February 28, 1928, Mahatma Gandhi returned
to the very plan he had adopted and discarded six years
before: a campaign of civil disobedience in the single district of Bardoli, in the Bombay Presidency. This time,
with careful preparation and with Sardar Vallabbhai
Patel in charge, it was to be a campaign to the end, for
the government had decreed a twenty-two-per-cent increase in taxation for the peasants of Bardoli, and they
could not pay it.

Gandhi stayed in his *ashram* most of this time and directed operations from afar. Patel, a brilliant Bombay
lawyer who had now been his follower for some twelve
years, was the field general for the struggle. It went on
from February 28 to August 6. The eighty-seven thousand peasants of Bardoli refused to pay their taxes. The
government fumed and raged. Cattle, carts, all possessions
were seized, many peasants went to jail, and still there
was no settlement. Land was taken, too, and a threat was
put forward at one time to sell it all to new peasants. The
peasants held firm, and what was more, there was no violence at all. Gandhi's wishes were obeyed in all things.

Money poured in from all over India to help the peasants keep alive and continue their struggle. Millions of
rupees were contributed by the rich Indians living abroad.
On June 12, when the struggle had been continuing for
three and a half months, Gandhi proclaimed a *hartal* for
all India in sympathy for Bardoli. Again, as once before,
India was completely paralyzed: nobody went to work
and no public service or commercial enterprise could
function. These immense warnings to the obdurate British were brought about with no violence whatsoever, in
perfect order and discipline.

On August 6 the government gave in, repealed the
twenty-two-per-cent increase in taxes, released the Bardoli prisoners, returned the confiscated land, and promised to make good on the animals or property that had
been seized.

The significance of the victory, promising greater vic-
tories on a larger scale whenever the Mahatma wished to
bring them about, was not lost on India. The whole
country now wanted to know what to do next. Talk of
complete independence was becoming common. "*Swaraj*," self-rule, was too vague a term for the young men.
Subhas Chandra Bose, then in the early stages of his career as a nationalist idol for the Bengal people, was a
frank believer in violence as a political weapon. Jawaharlal Nehru, though not bloodthirsty like Bose, was very
"advanced" in those days, and also wanted independence
as the declared aim of the nationalist movement.

Gandhi distrusted all this hotheadedness because he
feared that it might lead to violence, in which—aside
from his moral and religious scruples—he knew that the
dangers to India would be very great. He went to the

annual Congress meeting (Calcutta, December 1928) in a mood of caution, and did his best to discourage the young men. Talk of a declaration of independence seemed to him vain when it was by no means clear how such independence might be attained. The "war of independence" which was in the air (Bose's idea) was one that he could never have sanctioned. He was unable to put down the revolt of the young men at Calcutta, and compromised by asking for a delay of two years; when even this seemed too much to them, he cut it down to one year. If they would wait for one year he would join them: that is, if India had not attained *Swaraj* by the end of 1929, the Mahatma promised to support a declaration of complete independence. With this the young men had to be content.

Gandhi spent the year touring India, trying to prepare the people for a gigantic effort of *satyagraha* in the months to come. He did not talk politics much: he tried instead to explain his principles more and more clearly so that he might be able to count on truth and non-violence when the hour should strike. Meanwhile the elections in England had resulted in a coalition government with Ramsay MacDonald as Prime Minister and Wedgwood Benn at the India Office. The omens were a little better for India, and after a journey to London the Viceroy, Lord Irwin, made a statement favoring a "Round Table Conference" of British and Indian representatives to study Indian constitutional progress, with Dominion Status as the aim. This, however, produced a storm in London, and the position of the Labour party, governing without a majority, was much too weak to hold against the Tory thunder. The Viceroy was, in effect, disavowed, and when Gandhi and the other leaders went to see him on December 23 he was forced to tell them that he could give no pledges—he could not "prejudge" the decisions of the Round Table Conference.

This was, in effect, the real decision. Gandhi now had no recourse. He went to the annual meeting of the Indian National Congress and there accepted the principle of a declaration of independence—complete independence from the British-tie. That Congress meeting, at Lahore, was for the first time presided over by Jawaharlal Nehru, then just forty years of age. Gandhi retired to his *ashram* afterwards to write the Declaration of Independence of India, proclaimed on January 26, 1930.

CHAPTER SIX

THE SALT MARCH TO VICTORY

FROM the moment of the Declaration of Independence it was known throughout the world that Gandhi would soon engage in a new campaign against the government, but nobody knew what form it would take. Gandhi himself was at a loss, it seems, for some time. Whatever he did had to be non-violent, injuring no individual Englishman; it must be loyally notified in advance to the opponent and carried out with rigid discipline in every part of the country. These were now understood to be his principles, and he had a phalanx of devoted followers among the political classes (besides his own *ashram* disciples, that is) who knew what he wanted and could explain it to the people. The specific form of *satyagraha* to be offered was a problem. Gandhi studied the laws and pondered. When Tagore visited him early in the year and asked him what was coming, the Mahatma told the poet that he could not see any light in the darkness: the means eluded him.

They did not elude him for long. From February onward those who read *Young India* realized that the Mahatma's thoughts were dwelling on the Salt Laws. Salt was a British government monopoly in India; nobody could make it or buy it except from the government. Two articles in *Young India* analyzed the Salt Laws and their iniquity as an example of foreign rule, foreign exploitation. Anybody familiar with Gandhi's methods might have guessed that he intended in some way to use this legislation as the exemplar of tyranny, against which *satyagraha* would be offered. Then, on March 2, 1930, Gandhi wrote his famous letter to the Viceroy. Its first sentence announces the reason for the letter:

Dear Friend, Before embarking on Civil Disobedience and taking the risk I have dreaded to take all these years, I would fain approach you and find a way out.

The letter proclaims his central principle ("I cannot intentionally hurt anything that lives, much less human beings"), but then proceeds to indict the British administration for its exploitation of India. He asks the Viceroy "on bended knee" to consider these things and discuss them. If no discussion is possible, "on the eleventh day of this month I shall proceed with such co-workers of the Ashram as I can take, to disregard the provisions of the Salt Laws. . . . It is, I know, open to you to frustrate my design by arresting me. I hope that there will be tens of thousands ready, in a disciplined manner, to take up the work after me."

Lord Irwin was faced with a tremendous problem, and we can have no doubt that he relied heavily upon cablegrams to and from London. Ramsay MacDonald's coalition government had to consider the fact that a great part of the Labour party was openly in favor of independence, or at least Dominion status, for India. The world at large awaited with intense interest. The main question for Lord Irwin, a man of rare quality, was whether or not to arrest Gandhi. We do not know what his orders from London were. Obviously it was very dangerous to arrest Gandhi just then: if he went to jail, there was no telling how violent the coming movement might become. He alone was the guarantee of non-violence. And yet—and yet—not to arrest him was to court a great disaster. Ei-

ther way, the chances against Irwin's success in this matter were heavy.

Years later Lord Irwin (by then Lord Halifax) told
me that his personal regard for "the little man" (Gandhi)
had never faltered, and that "the little man" had never
once broken his word. Furthermore, as is well known,
Lord Halifax is a very religious man, and nobody could
possibly see Gandhi without realizing that he was almost
purely a religious phenomenon. The conflict in Halifax's own breast must have been painful, and yet when
the decision was made to try repression, he repressed with
all his might, exactly as if he believed that this would settle the question. In the immediate situation created by
Gandhi's letter, the Viceroy decided to side-step. He had
a secretary write the answer, which simply said that His
Excellency regretted to learn that Mr. Gandhi intended
to act in a way "clearly bound to involve violation of the
law and danger to the public peace."

Gandhi waited, prayed, meditated, while the whole
world (by then thoroughly on the alert) grew more at-
tentive to his slightest word. He had made it plain that
what he was going to do would involve violation of the
Salt Laws, but beyond this, nobody even in India knew
what was coming. His natural sense of drama, manifested
at all the great crises throughout his life, prompted him
to keep his own counsel until the great day arrived. On
that day, March 12, 1930, he and seventy-eight members of his *ashram* started out to walk from the neighborhood of Ahmedabad to a place called Dandi, on the
seacoast two hundred miles away. He had given the Viceroy an extra day of grace—the march began only on
the 12th.

By this time Sabarmati was besieged by the press of

the entire world, and by dense crowds of waiting Indians who wanted simply to know what the Mahatma was going to do. Much of the world-wide furor created by the Salt March arose from sheer curiosity, mixed with incredulity—the twentieth century could not quite believe such things even when they happened in the most relentless blaze of public attention.

On the morning of the 12th there were prayers and hymns in the *ashram*, and then the Mahatma set forth, followed by his seventy-eight disciples, men and women, and by great crowds that were forever changing but never absent. He went some of the time barefoot and some of the time in sandals. There was a horse along, throughout the march, for Gandhi's use in case he got tired, but he never used it. "We are marching in the name of God," he said.

The excitement throughout India has perhaps never been equaled. The Salt March lasted twenty-four days. The little old man in the loincloth was the center of the world's attention when he started out; by the time the Salt March ended, no other topic anywhere aroused such universal interest. Those twenty-four days brought the whole question of India's destiny into the sharpest focus it had ever had in the general view of mankind.

Gandhi was happy and healthy, as always when he was doing something he regarded as God's work. Some of his disciples grew sore and weary, but he never flagged. He thought twelve miles a day, the most they could manage in such a procession, no strain at all. At each village he would stop and talk to the people, telling them that a great ordeal was at hand, and that they must live purely, tell the truth, wear only homespun, wash themselves regularly, forswear alcohol and drugs, give up the abuses of

Hinduism (such as child marriage), and prepare to break the Salt Laws when the signal would be given them.

The people of India understood Gandhi as he understood them. They did not know what he was going to do, but they realized that it would be their signal. Printed words and even spoken words are as nothing against the power of a symbolic act, and it was Gandhi's genius, repeatedly throughout his life, to speak to his people without any words at all.

The villagers sprinkled the roads to keep the dust from his feet; they strewed leaves and branches in his path; they followed him to the next village before turning back home. The procession went on and on, involving immense numbers of people, while the government sat back, bewildered and already aghast at the power of this strange new movement.

On April 5, 1930, Gandhi and his immediate followers prayed all night long. In the early morning they went down to the sea. The Mahatma dipped into the water and picked up some salt from the shore. It was only a pinch of salt, but it was enough. He had broken the law and defied the Empire.

Salt was the commonest of necessities, and it had been monopolized by the foreign government. Salt was something every peasant could understand. Salt was God's gift, and the wicked foreign government had stolen it from the people. All this, and much more, went into the reverberant meanings of the act.

And, what is more, the disciplined execution of the salt campaign was the high point of *satyagraha* as a whole. Demonstrably it hurt nobody; it was perfectly non-violent; it was merely illegal. The government was compelled to act precisely as Gandhi had foreseen, and with the results he had foreseen.

The Mahatma himself was not arrested at once. The whole country burst into a flame of action as soon as the signal had been given on the seashore at Dandi. Everybody made salt, sold or bought salt, did everything possible to contravene the Salt Laws. The government resolutely began arresting people from one end of India to the other, but others constantly took their places. Neither the police nor the army could adequately deal with a situation in which virtually the whole population was breaking the law. Nor were the jails of India able to hold all the law-breakers, or even a sizable fraction of them. And all this without violence on the part of any Indian except in one isolated episode. The police and the soldiers were violent at times, but the people now had learned Gandhi's lesson and they did not even defend themselves.

Gandhi remained in camp with his seventy-eight followers for the weeks that followed. He did not again make salt or pick it up; there was no need for him to do so, as millions were doing it for him all along the immense seacoast of India. The Congress party organized the illegal sale of salt—illegal but quite public—on a great scale throughout the nation. Salt was sold for money which went into the party funds. The highest price was paid for the pinch of salt Gandhi had picked up on the beach: it fetched 1,600 rupees, perhaps $750 at the time. Mass meetings took place in all the cities, where illegal salt was sold and the boycott of foreign cloth was pledged. The government went on and on with the campaign of repression, until by the end of a single

month over sixty thousand persons were in jail for break-
ing the Salt Laws. Censorship was imposed on the Indian
press; the Congress papers simply ceased publication.
One by one the leaders of India went to jail, Nehru in
Allahabad, Rajagopalachari in Madras, Rajen Babu in
Patna, Devadas Gandhi in Delhi. On the night between
May 4 and 5, at forty-five minutes past midnight, Gan-
dhi was arrested.

This arrest was indeed curious: it was made under a
regulation of 1827 which had been in disuse for a very
long time. The warrant (or written order) merely said
that Mohandas Karamchand Gandhi was to be placed
under restraint and imprisoned "at the pleasure of the
Government." There was no charge and no trial. He
was taken to Yeravda Central Jail. There he was happy
with his spinning and letter-writing and his books.

The salt campaign continued. Gandhi had intended to
raid the Dharasana Salt Works, and had so informed the
Viceroy. This act was carried out by Sarojini Naidu,
whose radiant personality shines through the whole Gandhian epic and is forever to be remembered in India. The
well-known American correspondent Webb Miller was
present at the Dharasana raid and wrote a description of
it on the day itself. Twenty-five hundred volunteers advanced on the salt works in carefully chosen and orderly
detachments, one wave at a time. In front of the barbed-
wire stockade the police received them with steel-tipped
sticks (*lathis*). Sarojini Naidu had told them, after
prayers that morning, that they would be beaten but that
they must not resist: "You must not even raise a hand to
ward off a blow."

Webb Miller (as quoted by Fischer in his *Life of Mahatma Gandhi*) wrote:

Suddenly, at a word of command, scores of native police-men rushed upon the advancing marchers and rained blows on their heads with their steel-shod *lathis.* Not one of the marchers even raised an arm to fend off the blows. They went down like ten-pins. From where I stood I heard the sickening whack of the clubs on unprotected skulls. The waiting crowd of marchers groaned and sucked in their breath in sympathetic pain at every blow. Those struck down fell sprawling, unconscious or writhing with fractured skulls or broken shoulders. . . . The survivors, without breaking ranks, silently and doggedly marched on until struck down.

Later on he says:

The police commenced savagely kicking the seated men in the abdomen and testicles. [Later on:] Hour after hour stretcher-bearers carried back a stream of inert, bleeding bodies.

This astounding scene was repeated for several days thereafter, and on all these occasions the violence was en-tirely on the side of the police: no Gandhi follower made the slightest defense.

Sarojini Naidu got her accolade at Dharasana; she was arrested the first day. Motilal Nehru was arrested June 30 (he must have been anxious because they waited so long to do it—every patriot in India *wanted* to be ar-rested).

The government was in grave difficulty now; all work was handicapped to some extent by the resignations of numerous Indians in the offices; revenue was declining rapidly; the jails were packed (one hundred thousand political prisoners) and the police were weary; there seemed no issue from this dilemma except by giving in to Gandhi. Gandhi, when approached in Yeravda Jail, said he could not discuss terms without consulting members of the Congress Working Committee. The government then transported its most notable prisoners (by special train) to Yeravda Jail to talk with the Mahatma. The two Nehrus and Syed Mohammed were thus moved; Mrs. Naidu and Patel were both already in Yeravda Jail. In the result a communiqué was issued saying that an "unbridgeable gulf" separated these Indian leaders from the British on terms for peace.

There was a Round Table Conference on India in London in November 1930, but it was quite useless because no leader of consequence except Mohammed Ali Jinnah was able or willing to attend it. The time had come for the government to give in, and it did.

The Indian leaders, beginning with Gandhi, were set free on Indian Independence Day, January 26, 1931. No conditions were attached. The Mahatma wrote at once to the Viceroy, thanking him for this act and asking if they could not talk things over.

The Gandhi-Halifax (or Gandhi-Irwin) conversations had the historic importance of being the first in which Indian and Englishman spoke as equals, representing countries which henceforth would deal with each other as equals. The whole process of the liberation of India, which took seventeen more years to complete, was contained, essentially, in the Gandhi-Irwin conversations and the pact that was their outcome.

Winston Churchill saw this most clearly when he made his celebrated invective in the House of Commons, speaking of "the nauseating and humiliating spectacle of this one-time Inner Temple lawyer, now seditious fakir, striding half-naked up the steps of the Viceroy's palace, there to negotiate and to parley on equal terms with the representative of the King-Emperor."

Irwin, so tall, so infinitely *grand seigneur*, must indeed have made a striking contrast to the dark little man in the loincloth, whose greatness was of another kind, and whose unique demeanor treated everybody he met as an equal. This characteristic of Gandhi's was noticed and frequently described on his visit to London later in the year, but it was something rather new in the viceregal palace.

With Irwin, regardless of the surroundings, the Mahatma made good progress. They ended their series of conversations with a high mutual regard in spite of a great deal of hard, detailed bargaining and some long, weary disagreements. The first talk, lasting three and a half hours, took place on February 17, and was followed by others every day for a while; then came a week's interruption, and they returned to the task on February 27. Irwin was obliged to consult London at every stage, and Gandhi had to keep the Congress Working Committee fully informed and in agreement. On March 1, for example, Gandhi was at the palace all afternoon and again all evening, walking five miles each way, and when he got back to Dr. Ansari's house, where he was staying, the Working Committee was waiting for him (2:00 a.m.) for another session.

The Gandhi-Irwin Pact, signed March 7, 1930, made no stipulation on the future status of India. Gandhi stood on independence as the goal and said so; this agreement was "provisional" and "conditional." The Pact restored peace to India, in that civil disobedience would be called off, the political prisoners released, and salt made free along the seacoasts. Politically speaking, the chief historic gain was that the Indian National Congress agreed to be represented at the second Round Table Conference in London.

However, as Fischer and others have quite accurately pointed out, the Pact itself was more important than any of its contents. Its essential character is that of an agreement between equals, and in this respect it constitutes a tacit acknowledgment of independence. The seventeen transitional years that followed may have made many Indians impatient and caused others to doubt British good faith, but the main point was gained in 1930 and all the rest was detail.

Gandhi stood now at the apex of his career, politically speaking: he had liberated India by means not previously known or employed on any such scale. The annual meeting of the Congress elected him as its sole representative at the Round Table Conference in London, and he sailed on August 29.

2

The Round Table Conference brought Gandhi more squarely into the center of the whole world's attention than he had ever been. The press of the period, in all nations, reflects the intense curiosity he had aroused, though it does not always show the respect which those who came near him invariably felt. His clothing and diet, for example, commanded more space in the American press than his ideas. He could not alter his habits just because he was on a mission to the West. He traveled to England as a deck passenger, with his own goat, which he milked for his two principal meals. He would not go to a West End hotel in London, but stayed at Miss Muriel Lester's settlement house in the slums. This was so far from St.

James's Palace, the seat of the conference, that much time was consumed in transit, and for compromise an office was taken at 88 Knightsbridge. Gandhi went back to Kingsley Hall every night, just the same, because he liked to live among the poor.

And they liked him to be there. He was followed in the streets by friendly crowds, and often by children. It is much to the credit of the English character that in all this visit to England, in the midst of an outburst of public curiosity almost without precedent, nobody showed any open hostility to Gandhi—in fact few native-born English heroes have been so warmly greeted by the multitude. Quite a few detectives must have been scattered about in these crowds, but they had no work to do. What seems likely is that Gandhi's transparent honesty, his simplicity, and his evident friendliness toward all human creatures won the people's hearts and caused them to ignore the political differences that had brought him to London. Even in Manchester, which was in the midst of a terrible crisis of unemployment and depression brought about partly by his efforts, he was welcomed by cheering thousands.

The Gandhi legend, now in its full maturity, multiplied incessantly during these weeks and filled the press of the world with stories, some true and some false, but all more or less in character. He seems never to have protested against this spate of Gandhi stories—most of which he may not have heard—except for one: he denied that he had "prostrated himself" before the Prince of Wales during that dignitary's visit to India. Everybody of note and many of no note wanted a "Gandhi interview": scholars, theologians, and scientists as well as politicians or journalists. Bernard Shaw, the Archbishop of Canterbury, the King, the Queen, the youngest American newspaper reporter, the children in the streets—all were the same to Gandhi, and he treated them exactly alike. The loincloth, the goat, the almost toothless grin, the unfailing good humor, and the love of innocent laughter—all this became familiar to the whole Western world in such a wealth of detail as one can scarcely remember in any other connection.

One of the innumerable Gandhi jokes is still in my memory. It was a drawing in the *New Yorker* magazine, showing two ladies of the chorus in conference. One is saying to the other: "Why worry so much about clothes? Gandhi doesn't—and look at the publicity he gets!" His own remark on this subject, "You wear plus-fours and I wear minus-fours," went round the world. When an East End child called out at him in the streets: "Hey, Gandhi, where's your trousers?" the Mahatma's laughter was promptly cabled everywhere.

Gandhi's time in England (almost three months) was spent more in an effort to get the English people into sympathy with India than it was on the Round Table Conference itself. This, of course, he did attend, as the sole Congress representative, but there was little likelihood of a firm agreement because he was obliged at the outset to make it clear that the Congress wanted a complete independence for India. This was contrary to Article 2 of the Gandhi-Irwin Pact, which had reserved defense and foreign affairs, as well as national debts to foreigners, for British control. The Congress had repudiated Gandhi on this, and he was now under instructions to say so. To the English it seemed that the repudiation was Gandhi's; he had signed the Pact and now was going back on his own signature. In fact, as we can see now, it made no great difference. Independence was on the way, was im-

plicit in the entire proceeding, but the historic moment
for it had not arrived mainly because the British were not
yet ready for it. To Gandhi it was probably apparent that
he could not get complete independence for India then,
whatever he did, and that the best course would be to
prepare the English people to grant it in the future.

He talked incessantly to every kind of audience, visited
Oxford and Cambridge, Lancashire and Eton, and a
large number of organized groups in London. He said
with his usual candor that this was his real work: "The
seed which is being sown now may result in softening the
British spirit." His main effort was to explain the meaning of independence for India, and his definitions were
remarkably like what eventually took place. He would
cut India off "from the Empire entirely, from the British
nation not at all, if I want India to gain and not to grieve.
The Emperorship must go and I should love to be an
equal partner with Britain, sharing her joys and sorrows,
and an equal partner with the Dominions. But it must be
a partnership on equal terms." This was to be, "if God
wills it, an indissoluble partnership, but not a partnership
superimposed upon one nation by another . . . England and India should be bound by the silken cord of
love."

Gandhi's work was not confined to Indians; its effects
were deeply felt in England, and when independence did
come, its form was freely decided by both sides—that is,
England freely and unconditionally granted it, and India
one year later chose to remain in "association" with the
Commonwealth as an independent Republic. This was,
from both the British and the Indians, a precise fulfillment of Gandhi's plea in 1930. It required, however,
the free grant of independence as a prerequisite to part-

nership, an act of gift from England. In conversation
with Edgar Snow not long before his death, the Mahatma
actually used the word "gift"—"since the English have
made us this great gift."

The Round Table Conference itself, as a body to
plan India's future, started with hardly any chance of
success, as it was composed of inherently divisive elements. Lord Reading, at the outset, defined its purpose
as being "to give effect to the views of India while preserving at the same time our own position, which we
must not and cannot abandon." There were among the
Indians present twenty-three princes or their representatives, and sixty-four representatives from British India,
of whom only Gandhi and a very few of his friends represented the mass movement of the Congress. The Viceroy
(now Lord Willingdon) had sent to London a hand-
picked collection of reactionaries and fractional representatives whose ideas, training, and interests were all against
any form of real union in India. Each fraction wanted to
vote separately, as a fraction—Moslems voting for Moslems, Parsees for Parsees, and so on—in the legislative
elections to be set up under the new constitution.

This was contrary to every principle or wish Gandhi
had. He wanted no separate electorates—Indians were all
Indians and should vote as Indians. The perpetuation of
India's divisions would, he foresaw, lead to more and
greater trouble. In spite of his unique authority and prestige, he was so greatly outnumbered at this conference
that his views had no chance of prevailing. He attended
all the meetings, sitting usually with his eyes closed, but
so much of the discussion was purely political (political
on a fairly low level) that it may be his mind did not
receive everything his ears heard. He meditated a good

deal and may also have slept a little. Conferences, like legislatures, were not his element; he liked to talk as an individual to individuals.

The conference ended on December 1, 1931, in complete failure. By dividing the Indians more sharply than ever before, it probably made things a good deal worse. It has been suggested that this was, indeed, the British purpose—*divide et impera*—but one can hardly attribute such conscious duplicity to Ramsay MacDonald, whose benevolence, at that period, so greatly surpassed his intellect. No: rather it seems, in retrospect, that many of the British claims for protection of the Indian sovereign princes, or for protection of "minorities" (Moslem, Parsee, Christian, Anglo-Indian, considering Hindus to be the "majority") were real. That is, the British representatives at the conference, who numbered twenty, were for the most part convinced that they had a genuine duty toward all these fractions in India. Underneath all that, there probably was also the tenacious hope that Britain somehow could hang on to India, glory and profits alike, but it is a characteristic of Anglo-Saxon governments on both sides of the Atlantic to find noble reasons for self-interest.

What saddened Gandhi most, one must infer, is the imputation in all this that he and his friends, representing the great majority in India, were not to be trusted—that if they had their way the "minorities" would be bound to suffer. Every effort Gandhi himself had made toward Hindu-Moslem unity and the reconciliation of all races, castes, and creeds was thus treated as insignificant. This in itself need not have troubled him, as he had no wish to be credited with any achievement, but it was unquestionably apparent to him that by acting as they did, the

British jeopardized the chances for such unity and reconciliation in the future. British prestige was, in spite of
everything, high in India (as it still is), and nothing
could be easier for a factional agitator from then on than
to claim British support or approval. It was this danger
to the future rather than the immediate failure of the conference that weighed on Gandhi's spirit. He had expected
nothing much from the conference, and had indeed said
on leaving India that he would probably come back
empty-handed, but the result was worse than he had
anticipated.

3

On his way to Bombay, Gandhi stopped in Lausanne
to have his celebrated series of conversations with Romain
Rolland, most of which have been published in various
forms. They discussed principles rather than events, and
found themselves in essential accord. Rolland, who had
written a biography of Gandhi seven years before, had
never met him, and had in fact never been to India,
though his interest had been shown in his work. It is
pleasant to reflect that when Gandhi (who cared not a
great deal for either art or music) asked Rolland to play
the piano, the French writer, whose devotion to music
was profound, gave him the *andante* from Beethoven's
Fifth Symphony.

The Mahatma also stopped in Rome, where he was
obliged to spend a fruitless twenty minutes talking to
Benito Mussolini. The person he actually wished to see
was the Pope, but the Vatican, having just put its relations with Great Britain on a new and friendlier basis,
did not see fit to grant his request. Mr. Winston Church-

ill and Pius XI were thus the only persons of whom we have record who refused a conversation with Gandhi.

His return to Bombay was triumphal from the point of view of public demonstrations, but the news he learned at disembarkation was anything but good. The government had started a new campaign of repression and arrests in the north and northwest because of a Congress campaign against paying rent. Jawaharlal Nehru had been put in jail two days before Gandhi's homecoming. Gandhi tried at once to see the Viceroy (Lord Willingdon), but the exchange of telegrams was very stiff; the Viceroy obviously did not want to see him. The homecoming was December 28, 1931; and on January 4, 1932, the Mahatma was arrested again. This time, as the time before, no charges were made and no trial was held; he was in Yeravda Jail at the government's pleasure.

He was, as we know, always happy in jail, but he can hardly have failed to grin his snaggle-toothed best when he reflected how recently he had been a popular hero to the British people and an honored guest of their King and Queen. However, his usual jail happiness was impaired and finally extinguished by the decision of the British government to create, in the new constitution for India, separate electorates not only for Hindus and Moslems, but also for the "Depressed Classes," the untouchables. For these people, the stepchildren of Hinduism, Gandhi had labored all his life, but he did not want them used as a means of dividing Indians from one another. He wrote first to Sir Samuel Hoare, the Secretary of State for India (March 11) and finally to Ramsay MacDonald, the Prime Minister (August 18). Between March and August the British government had plenty of time to grow more familiar with his views, which were available not only in his letters, but also in numerous printed forms. Nevertheless they went on with the scheme, which MacDonald announced in London on August 17.

Gandhi's response was terrible. He declared (August 18) in his letter to MacDonald that he would be compelled to fast "unto death," beginning September 20.

A good many Indians of Western education were as puzzled by Gandhi's fast this time as Ramsay Mac-Donald was. MacDonald wrote a long, earnest letter trying to remove Gandhi's "misapprehension" of the special treatment for untouchables. Gandhi's reply was that this, to him, was a matter of religion, and that his prayer would be to "sting the Hindu religious conscience." He was not fasting *against* the British government, but to arouse the Hindus themselves to their religious duty.

The fast began on September 20 at noon. Many millions of Indians fasted on that day; prayers were offered everywhere; the country was in mourning. Gandhi seems to have cared for Tagore's opinion more than for that of anybody else at the critical moment, and Tagore—not always a blind follower—sustained him with wonderful words of praise and comprehension. Tagore's explanation of the "self-immolation" of Gandhi is eloquent: he says: "The penance which Mahatmaji has taken upon himself is not a ritual but a message to all India and to the world."

The Indian leaders hastily began to negotiate some kind of settlement which would induce Gandhi to cease fasting. He was not strong at this time, and even the first twenty-four hours visibly sapped his reserves. On the fourth day he was thought to be sinking, and serious fear for his life fell upon the whole country. Ambedkar, the untouchable leader, who was not a Gandhi follower, was the most difficult for the Hindus to deal with, and yet no compromise settlement would be worth making unless it bore his signature. He visited Gandhi in jail, and the general lines of an agreement were approved by the Mahatma; it was hammered out in long, labored discussions of all the leaders and signed by them on September 24. The Mahatma was not, of course, a signatory, but he approved of the compromise; he could not cease fasting until the British government had also approved.

MacDonald, Hoare, Lothian, and others who had scattered for the week-end returned to London that Sunday (September 25) and studied the text of the Yeravda Pact, as it is called, until midnight. On Monday it was simultaneously announced in London and Delhi that the British government would accept the Pact. The Mahatma's fast ended that day, when he accepted a glass of orange juice from Kasturbai.

This was by no means his longest fast, but it seems to have had a more damaging effect on him than any other. He was actually on the point of death, by the doctors' opinions, for the last two days of it. One is tempted to offer the hypothesis, for what it is worth, that the mere fact of its being a fast "unto death" introduced into the Mahatma's consciousness the idea of death, thus, for a creature made up mostly of mind and spirit, impairing the strength of his fragile little body. No fast before now had been declared "unto death," and in fact Gandhi had a religious and ethical horror of suicide as a great sin. The probability is that his profound instinctive knowledge of his own people assured him that they would not let him die, but would at all costs compose their differences; but

this knowledge was crossed by the thought that he was
growing old and that the words "unto death" were very
solemn words.

At all events, the fast had an electrical effect on Indian
society. In demonstrations throughout the country, in
cities or in villages, caste Hindus mingled with untouchables, accepted food from their hands, and ate meals with
them; large numbers of temples and holy places were
thrown open to the pariahs; pledges to work against discrimination were made on an enormous scale and sent to
Gandhi's prison. The six days of the fast were treated as
a period of mourning throughout India, and the end of
the fast was the occasion for national celebration.

Gandhi had asked the Hindu mind to "banish untouchability root and branch." For this larger objective
the agreement on a combined electorate was not in itself
very important, but the great movement throughout
Hindu society to meet Gandhi's wishes was a vital force,
and goes on today. Nobody pretends that untouchability,
a very ancient abuse, can quickly go, but nobody can
deny that an effort in that direction has been and is being
made. The Mahatma's most permanent objective, the
"purification of India," which always seemed to him
more important than anything in politics, was advanced
by the fast of 1932 more than by decades of preaching
or teaching.

And, too, it seems to have turned the Mahatma's own
mind more firmly toward those non-political purposes
which commanded his adherence. He referred to these
purposes, in conversation with me, as "my constructive
work," perhaps with the implication that anything done
in a political way was not really constructive. From the
fast on until the outbreak of the Second World War,

Gandhi left politics to others and spent most of his time and energy on his work for the untouchables, for women and children in the villages, for "Basic Education," and for the spinning-wheel. These were activities which, like nursing the sick, appealed to his innermost nature. He could walk from village to village barefoot, week after week and month after month with apparently indefatigable energy, preaching against untouchability, telling the people to be clean and to love one another. And at the outset of this period, for "self-purification," he undertook a fast of twenty-one days. On the day it began, the government released him from prison, as his death there would have been a calamity for the British Raj. It did not seem possible that he could survive a fast of three whole weeks, when only six days of abstinence from food had brought him to death's door six months earlier. And yet the long fast, unaccompanied by the anxiety of the six days in September, left him as well as ever—he would have said, better.

He founded the Harijan Sevak Sangh, a society to improve the lot of the untouchables by model villages and schools and in other ways, in February 1933, while he was still in prison, and at the same time started a weekly paper called *Harijan* to take the place of *Young India*. *Harijan* was his own word for the untouchables; it means "Children of God." From that time until his death he never ceased to do everything he could, in the most practical way, for these oppressed victims of the caste system. His model villages for Harijans were clean and attractive; his schools were adapted to Indian conditions; and he never ceased to collect money for them. One of his endearing habits in later years was to give his autograph—which was constantly in demand—in ex-

change for five or ten rupees for the Harijan work. Anybody who wrote to him, from any part of the world,
could get the signature, but he firmly collected the fee.

Basic education and the work for villagers (especially
women) were among Gandhi's "constructive" efforts.
His ideas of "Basic Education" were in conformity with
Indian conditions and have been carried out on a very
large scale in several provinces since his death. He had
been much impressed by Mme Montessori and her
methods in London in 1930, and his own system may
owe a good deal to her. He started, as always, with the
mass level, the level of the poor Indian villager whose
maintenance standards (food and clothing) he emulated.
Such a villager cannot afford to lose the work of his children. Therefore the school must combine learning with
useful work, which should be remunerated. (This element was much criticized, and I think very stupidly, as
leading to "child labor"—which, with or without school-
ing, is a commonplace in India anyhow.) That is, if a
boy can make a good bench or a pair of sandals he ought
to be paid for them, and his school time must be appor-
tioned between useful arts of this sort and ordinary
learning. The system of "Basic Education," as it is called,
is far more developed than I have indicated, but this is its
essential character.

Gandhi in his unceasing movement about India
brought all his ideas to the people as nobody, in all probability, since Gautama Buddha. It is quite possible to find
places in India which Gandhi never visited—the country
is enormous and the villages are practically innumerable
—but they are not many. Almost any Indian one meets
anywhere, including the poorest, has a memory of at
least one sight of the Mahatma. At Almora in the Hima-

layan foothills, where I visited the local jail (mainly because it was Mr. Nehru's prison at one time), a prisoner
talking to me through the bars told me he had followed
the Mahatma on part of the Salt March. A maharajah
may say: "I saw him in 1934," and an untouchable may
say: "I saw him once in Madras," but neither could
possibly forget it.

4

Gandhi was "out of politics," as the expression goes,
but in fact he could never really remove himself from
that realm or from any other in Indian life. Politicians
were forever consulting him about questions big and
little; he would not scruple to make them wait outside
while he doctored a beggar or administered to a leper.
His scale of values was not theirs, and yet they could not
go on without him. His approval was necessary for any
decision of importance, and his disapproval was fatal to
any idea, career, or activity. Jawaharlal Nehru, recur-
rently president of the Congress, said that Gandhi was
"the permanent Super-President." When Gandhi consented to Indian participation in the legislatures set up
under the new constitution, Congress candidates were
triumphant in many provinces and took part in the government. This was, in Gandhi's eyes, a prelude to independence, perhaps a training for it. He did not himself
take part, and it is said that he only once visited a legislature, and that as a guest in the public gallery.

The Second World War was the occasion of his return to public affairs. When war was declared, the British
government brought India into it at once without consulting any Indian person. This offended all opinion in
India, particularly that of the political classes and per-

sonalities. The Viceroy (by this time it was Lord Linlithgow) asked Gandhi to come to Simla on the day
after the war was declared, and the Mahatma went.

In the Simla interview Gandhi and Linlithgow talked
sadly of war's inevitable destruction, and Gandhi's natural
sympathy (indeed his love) for England came into full
play. He had watched the progress of Fascism in Europe
with much foreboding, and he was quite clear in his con-
demnation of Hitler's system: it was "naked ruthless
force reduced to an exact science and worked with scientific precision." He pledged his moral support to England
and the allies, and declared that "my whole heart is with
the Poles in the unequal struggle in which they are engaged for the sake of their freedom."

These declarations were as far as he would go in sup-
porting the war; he did not intend to take any active part
and would not even have defended India against aggression. Thus he was out of step with both the British and
the Indian political leaders. The Congress point of view
was that India could support the war effort on certain
political conditions. Gandhi was never willing to bargain
on a principle, and in this case his central principles were
directly at issue. "Whatever support was to be given to
the British should be given unconditionally," he said.
Nevertheless the Congress political leaders went ahead
with their manifesto of September 14, 1939, which con-
demned Hitler's aggression but also blamed the Western
democracies for their imperialism and concluded that "a
free India" would gladly associate itself with other free
nations. This manifesto (the work of Jawaharlal Nehru)
did not represent Gandhi's views at all, but once it had
been issued he asked the country to support it. His reason
for doing so was that his "best co-workers" wanted it and

he could not desert them, but only must hope that "their departure from the non-violent method will be confined to the narrowest field and will be temporary."

The Viceroy in replying to the Congress manifesto said, obviously on orders from London, that England could not yet define war aims; he cautioned India against too rapid advances in self-government. The Congress thereupon voted to abstain from any help to England, and asked the Congress members of provincial governments to resign.

Gandhi's delicate conscience at this period seems to have been walking fearfully over some extremely fragile eggshells. He did not like to have even the appearance of taking advantage of England's difficulties, and he disliked having to disagree with the "best co-workers," probably Nehru most of all. Above all, he wished to cling, more than ever before, to the principle of non-violence. Meanwhile the rush of events in the spring of 1940 threw India, too, like most of the world, into apprehension; Hitler seemed to have conquered Europe. There was some panic, some runs on British banks. Gandhi asked the country to be calm and said that if Britain had to die, it would be "heroically." He seems to have had a very accurate notion of the last-ditch courage and essential toughness of the British people.

Nehru, however, in his desire both to aid the war effort and to get some advantage for India out of doing so, was in control of the Congress Working Committee, ably assisted by Rajagopalachari. Gandhi's non-violence did not suit the mood of the moment, and the Mahatma knew it. If he had insisted against all opposition, he probably could have forced the Working Committee to obey his will, but this was also contrary to his principle of non-violence and would have troubled his conscience. Under the circumstances, all he could do was let the vote decide, as it did—Rajaji's resolution (backed also by Nehru) was passed, and the Congress promised to "throw its full weight" into the defense effort if India was given independence and an Indian government.

Winston Churchill was Prime Minister in London, and the independence of India was never an acceptable idea to him. Quite aside from that fact, it may be historically doubted whether the crisis of a desperate war was the correct moment for such a difficult operation as the transfer of power. The transfer proved difficult enough when it did occur, seven years later; one shudders to think of what the results might have been in 1940.

In any case, the answer to Congress was a firm negative, accompanied by the statement that Britain could not yield power to an Indian government to which large sections of the Indian population objected. This was a reference to the non-Congress and anti-Congress Moslems, who had been organized into a new and vital opposition by Mohammed Ali Jinnah.

Congress now swayed in the direction of non-violent non-cooperation again. It must have been all too evident to Gandhi that the political leaders adopted his principles when they thought it advantageous to do so, or when there was nothing else they could do, but were willing to abandon them with equal fervor. Nevertheless, the Mahatma welcomed them back on his side, but cautioned them against doing anything to embarrass the British. He went in behalf of the Congress to see the Viceroy, proposing that the Congress should be free to work among the people even though it would not support the war effort. This, too, was refused.

The shoals and whirlpools of Gandhi's conscience could not permit him to do any real harm to the British at such a moment, but neither could he accept this total denial of any rights to India. India had been dragged into the war without any consultation whatever, and was now to be gagged for the duration. Gandhi decided upon a small-scale campaign of disobedience, limited more or less to Congress leaders. He asked Vinoba Bhave to go to jail first, Nehru next, Patel next, and Maulana Abul Kalam Azad next. The Congress Working Committee had asked and obtained Gandhi's pledge that he would himself stay out of jail. In something like a year 23,223 persons were jailed for speaking against the war effort or the war itself.

Japan's entry into the war at the end of 1941 brought this phase of India's war experience to an end. The British government released the prisoners; Gandhi's views were no longer in control of Congress; he retired again from any participation in its debates; the Japanese army and navy were sweeping across southeast Asia and might soon be in India.

However, the United States and Russia were both now aligned against Hitler, and the United States against Japan as well. There was no longer any real doubt in high quarters that eventual victory was assured. But American opinion, always rather pro-Indian, was not happy over England's treatment of India; it seemed too much at variance with the declared purposes of the war. Much evidence has appeared in recent years to show that President Roosevelt never let the subject of India drop for long in his correspondence with Mr. Churchill. Strong elements in England itself agreed with Roosevelt rather than with Churchill: the Indian contradiction, it

seemed fairly plain, would have to be solved sooner or
later, and the sooner the better for Allied purposes.

It was at this point that Churchill sent Sir Stafford
Cripps to India with the idea of discussing possible constitutional changes with Indian leaders. Cripps had been
in India once before (in the preceding November), and
had visited Gandhi at the Wardha *ashram*. Now (March
22, 1942) he arrived in New Delhi with definite proposals for Dominion status. (Dominion status, since the
Westminster Statute of 1926, includes the right to leave
the Commonwealth at any time.) This was to come
when the war was over, and was to be accompanied by a
provision allowing any province or area that wished to do
so to secede from the Indian Union and form a separate
Dominion.

The only thing in the Cripps proposals that Gandhi
could have accepted was Dominion status. The rest—
special status for the Indian princes and the threat of
"vivisection"—he could not accept. The final article,
on the war effort, was antipathetic to his principles of
non-violence. Consequently Gandhi rejected the whole
Cripps proposal at first sight and went home to Wardha,
having nothing further to do with the negotiation.

Nehru and Rajaji continued the talks, as did the
leaders of many Indian factions and minorities, but in
the end all made the same reply—the proposals were
not acceptable. Cripps went back to England on April
12, the very day of Roosevelt's long cable pleading with
Churchill to try again. Churchill, obviously, had already
gone so far beyond his own true convictions in this matter that he must, one feels, have been glad that the Cripps
mission failed; the "dissolution of His Majesty's empire,"
as he called it, was for others to bring into history.

It will be a matter of debate, like so many other ifs, whether the immediate independence of India in 1942, at the time of the Cripps mission, would have saved India the ordeal that came five years later. Louis Fischer advances the theory that the transfer of power to an Indian government could have taken place in 1942 in an orderly manner because of the presence of British and allied troops, and that "real power" would have remained in British hands for the duration of the war. Yet it seems to me that if "real power" remained with the British, Gandhi would not have approved, and without his approval it could not have been done. Moreover, the Moslem separatist movement led by Mohammed Ali Jinnah was already very powerful and would have given great difficulty in 1942, as at any later time.

Perhaps Gandhi himself thought that the war period was the best time for Indian independence, but for a characteristically Gandhian reason—he wished to face the threatened Japanese invasion with a passive resistance on a mammoth scale, and could only do so if India was free to make the attempt. Without freedom, without a national government, India would of course be defended by British and allied forces in the conventional manner, and though Gandhi did not wish to impede them, neither would he aid them. It is evident that he had very seriously and thoroughly considered the situation that a Japanese invasion would present, and to his mind it would have been the greatest challenge ever offered to the efficacy of non-violent non-cooperation. Through 1942 he kept on telling Indians that this might take place and that they must have no dealings whatsoever with the invader.

Gandhi's thinking was far different from that of his

closest political friends and followers, all of whom wanted independence precisely so that they could fight the war. Nehru, in particular, was temperamentally unsuited to non-violence on the scale Gandhi had in mind. He had been an anti-Fascist for years, and wanted to fight "in every way possible," he said. Rajaji and the Maulana Sahib were of much the same cast of mind, though less passionate in expression. The prerequisite was immediate independence for India, and the Working Committee so resolved at Wardha on July 14. If this was refused, the resolution declared, the Congress would be "reluctantly compelled" into a campaign of civil disobedience.

The final decision was taken by the All-India Congress Committee meeting in Bombay, August 7–8, 1942. In Gandhi's mind it did not mean that civil disobedience should begin at once; he wanted, as usual, to try negotiation first, and intended to go to Delhi to see the Viceroy. He was actually working on a letter to President Roosevelt when he was arrested, very late that night (morning of August 9), and taken to his last prison, the palace of the Aga Khan at Poona. With him were also arrested most of the other Congress leaders.

These arrests ended any hope of a peaceful, non-violent campaign of civil disobedience. The Indian people were now leaderless and did not have the calming power of Gandhi's voice and example to deter them from excesses. Gandhi was kept without newspapers during the first part of his imprisonment, and actually did not know, except from his jailers, what was going on in the country. Yet the government evidently expected him to condemn and disavow it.

Bands of Indians were tearing up railroad tracks, engaging in sporadic acts of violence, cutting telegraph wires and attacking policemen. In some districts the movement, now completely out of hand, wore the aspect of armed rebellion.

Gandhi had never hesitated to condemn and disavow violence. In this case he did not wish to do so because he had only a "one-sided version" of what had taken place, and he had no means of investigating the truth for himself. Moreover, when he began receiving newspapers again, he could see that the governments both in Delhi and in London were engaged in what he called "distortions and misrepresentations," the purport of which was to make the Mahatma (or the Mahatma and the Congress) responsible for the disorder in India. It was a typical effort of war propaganda, and he resented it very much. Therefore his first letter to the Viceroy (August 14) from jail was not much like Gandhi; it was five pages long and filled with accusations. Linlithgow replied very briefly that he could not accept this criticism. One's guess is that he would not, himself, have arrested Gandhi without having a talk with him first; the peremptory course adopted must have originated in London.

On New Year's Eve, Gandhi again wrote to the Viceroy and said that he was hurt that such an old friend should have jailed him without a hearing. He said that he was not responsible for the violence in the country, but that the government itself was. He had decided to fast.

The Viceroy replied as soon as he saw the letter—but it had been fourteen days in getting to him. He was very depressed that Gandhi had not spoken to the people, condemning the violence and crime that were afoot.

Gandhi replied that he deplored the happenings in India, but could neither influence nor control them, and that he "laid the blame at the door of the Government of

India." Linlithgow replied that Gandhi and the Congress must bear the blame.

Gandhi replied by announcing a fast beginning February 9 and lasting twenty-one days.

The Viceroy wrote back immediately, reiterating that the Congress was responsible for the public disorder, hoping the Mahatma would not fast, and then stating with unusual bluntness: "I regard the use of a fast for political purposes as a form of political blackmail for which there is no moral justification, and understood from your own previous writings that this was also your view."

This was very strong language, considering how careful the Mahatma had always been to define his fasts. In his reply he said: "Despite your description of it as 'a form of political blackmail,' it is on my part an appeal to the Highest Tribunal for justice which I have failed to secure from you. If I do not survive the ordeal I shall go to the Judgment Seat with the fullest faith in my innocence. Posterity will judge between you as a representative of an all-powerful government and me a humble man who has tried to serve his country and humanity through it."

The government tried to get out of this dilemma by releasing Gandhi from prison, but he refused to be released. If released, he said, he would not fast—thus implying that he might engage in some other activity. He was just as troublesome to the Viceroy in jail as out of it, but it was thought safer to let him proceed to the fast while still confined. He was authorized to get any doctors or friends he wished to help him through the ordeal; there was plenty of room for all of them at the Aga Khan's palace.

This fast (February 10 to March 2, 1943) was a terrible one for everybody in India, and the government was in fairly continuous hot water from all directions. It became necessary to allow the crowds to pass through the palace and see the Mahatma with their own eyes, the fear of his death having gripped the country. He was sinking steadily after the first week, and it seems to have been universally expected that he would die before the twenty-one days were over. Kasturbai herself seems to have thought so. The bulletins were signed by British official doctors as well as by Gandhi's own, and they were not encouraging. The results for British relations with India were as bad as possible.

Gandhi's own unhappiness during the period in the Aga Khan's palace—August 1942–May 1944—was extreme. He had always loathed violence, and now it was rampant over India, officially ascribed to his own doings. If he had not been arrested, he felt, and arrested without any sort of hearing, he might have prevented the outbreak. Whatever civil-disobedience campaign he had chosen to undertake would have been of a non-violent character, and he had proved in the Salt March that it could be done. However, the government had been unwilling to wait or even to hear him.

To this daily misery two great personal griefs were now added one after the other—first, the death of his devoted secretary, Mahadev Desai, who had worked with him on his *Gita*; second, the death of Kasturbai herself, his lifelong companion, the wife of his youth. The Mahatma's sorrow in both cases was extreme, but he tried to express it in the *Gita* terms of detachment—not, perhaps, with much success. He had been living with Kasturbai at this time for sixty-two years, and although she, as a

devout and simple Hindu woman, had never been able
to follow him in all his experiments with truth, above all
in matters touching the caste system and ritual, she had
absorbed much of his teaching without question. Both
Mahadev and Kasturbai were cremated in the prison
courtyard and their ashes were buried side by side in the
grounds.

After this personal tragedy the Mahatma suffered two
severe illnesses, first malaria and afterwards an intestinal
trouble. The great Bengal famine of 1943 had come and
gone while he was in prison; the disaffection of the Indian
masses toward British rule was stronger than ever; it became obvious that if he died in prison very serious results
would probably ensue. The new Viceroy, Lord Wavell,
released Gandhi, Patel, Mrs. Naidu, and their associates
on May 6, 1944.

5

The story of the next three years is essentially the tale
of Gandhi's last struggle to save India from what he
called "vivisection." He had always worked toward national unity and against all the divisive tendencies (he
called them "fissiparous") in the vast sub-continent.
There now appeared on the horizon, just when the liberation of India was at hand, the most serious of all threats
to India's unity, a militantly nationalistic Moslem movement aiming at the creation of a separate nation.

That movement was recent: the very name of the new
nation, Pakistan, had not yet become generally known
or used. Moslems and Hindus had lived in all parts of
India for centuries, mixed together in the villages and
usually also in the towns. They were substantially the
same people, and most Moslems were descendants of

Hindus who had been converted to Islam at various periods (and usually by the sword) in previous centuries. The languages of the south were the same for Hindu and Moslem alike. In the north a language distinction existed between Urdu, the Moslem language written in its own script with strong Persian influences, and Hindi, written in its own script with strong Sanskrit influences; and yet even these two languages used to be quite close together and mutually intelligible.

Gandhi could see no reason why a separate Moslem state had to be: his famous expression on the subject, used to Mohammed Ali Jinnah, was: "You can cut me in two if you wish but don't cut India in two." Jinnah, on the contrary, declared that the Moslem nation already existed and must have its rights. One hundred million Moslems in a nation ruled by three hundred million Hindus would be submerged, he said. All the rest of the story up to the day of liberation is the story of this antagonism, this negotiation at times, this impossibility of negotiation at others.

Gandhi tried very hard. He knew, as he slowly recovered from his illness, that independence must be near, and could perhaps come now if he could unite the Moslems and the Hindus. Long years before, in South Africa, he had foreseen and stated that the "crucial test" would be this. As soon as he was able to do so, he wrote to Mohammed Ali Jinnah and proposed to talk over a compromise proposal.

Those conversations took place in Jinnah's fine house in Bombay during the summer of 1944, and were accompanied by long letters between the two, recapitulating what had been said in talk. The letters were afterwards published in full—after the breakdown of negotiations, that is—and they exhibit an extreme intransigence on Jinnah's part. He wanted the areas of big Moslem population to vote on secession from the Indian Union, but only Moslems should take part in such a vote: this meant that in a number of key provinces, where Moslems and Hindus were almost equal in population, the Hindus should be disenfranchised altogether. Gandhi was prepared, for the sake of peace, to let units of predominantly Moslem population vote for secession if they wished to do so after independence, but he hoped for a common administration in foreign affairs, customs, and the like.

Jinnah, an extremely able and sucessful lawyer, had once been a vigorous Congress party worker, but after a stay of some years in London had returned to India convinced that the Moslem League, once allied to the Congress, should take the field against it. His own personal jealousy of Gandhi's unique position may have had something to do with this, along with his great dislike for Jawaharlal Nehru. He was vain, as anybody knows who ever talked to him, and one element in his character must have been an unwillingness to play second fiddle to anybody—especially as he was quite honestly convinced of his own superiority. He made a militant anti-Congress force out of the Moslem League and adopted the Pakistan idea (which dates from 1936) as his war-cry. In this new state he wished to put the provinces of Sind, Baluchistan, the Punjab, the Northwest Frontier Province, Bengal, and Assam, with their existing boundaries, and consequently, of course, a huge Hindu minority that thus would have nothing to say about its own fate. In less than ten years Jinnah had transformed the whole situation in India, so that to most of the politically conscious and active Indians it appeared that the antagonist in the arena was not the British at all, but the Indians of another religion.

Lord Wavell called all the leaders to Simla at the end of June 1945, when Churchill was still Prime Minister, and put before them a scheme that would have made the Viceroy's Council entirely Indian, made up of Indians chosen by the Viceroy from lists drawn up by all parties. Moslems and Hindus were to be represented in "equal proportions," though Hindus outnumbered Moslems three to one. In effect, this was self-government, preserving only a vestige of the old Empire, and the Congress leaders were prepared to accept it. Jinnah refused. His main reason seems to have been that Wavell had named Moslem members of the Council, whereas he alone should have had that right. (The Congress, which had many Moslem members, had no right at all in his eyes.)

Events moved fast thereafter. Churchill was defeated in the British elections; a Labour government came to power and called Wavell home. On his return to India he announced a new plan, by which elections would be held for the provincial and central legislatures as a prelude to a new constitution. The elections resulted as might have been foreseen: Congress won in districts with Hindu majorities and the Moslem League won in Moslem areas.

To solve the problem of this tug-of-war, when Jinnah refused to budge from any position taken, was beyond the power of any element at hand in India. Gandhi had failed and said so; he did not take the course so many Indians preferred: blaming the British. Clement Attlee decided to send three members of his cabinet to India —the Cabinet Mission—with authority to draw up a scheme for the transfer of power from British to Indian hands. The Cabinet Mission consisted of Cripps, Pethick-

Lawrence, and A. V. Alexander, and they spent some two months in New Delhi and elsewhere, talking to Indian leaders, before they published their decisions on May 16, 1946.

The Mission had studied the ground carefully and had taken full account of Jinnah's demand for a separate Moslem nation. The report goes into that question in some detail, and points out that any line drawn for the partition of India would leave large minorities on each side, whereas lines drawn through the middle of provinces would violate local geography, economics, and traditions. In consequence, instead of partition, the Ministers recommended a federal government with majorities of both Moslems and Hindus required for anything that concerned the religious communities. An interim government was to prepare the way for a constituent assembly.

There was a period of uncertainty, in Gandhi's mind as in others, about these proposals: Gandhi himself was always ready to trust British intentions when they were clearly shown, but his instinct, apparently, was not clear about the present situation. In some important conversations he had with Louis Fischer at just this time he made it plain that he felt he had failed in his main mission in India—that Indians had not understood non-violence and therefore he could not take up any kind of civil-disobedience campaign again. He thought the best thing for the Congress leaders to do would be to go into the constituent assembly and make the best of it. His sadness about violence in India was shown many times in these talks, as in his written work of the period.

Gandhi had been consulted at every turn, of course, not only by the Congress leaders, but by the British as well. He was never a delegate or a member of any committee, but nothing in India could be done without his approval or at least consent. He was at this time not even a member of the Congress—"not even a four-anna member," he used to say, referring to the annual dues paid by members.

The uncertainty lasted well into 1946. Jinnah might have entered the provisional government, but refused because he would allow no Moslem except one of his own to be in it; Congress, too, had Moslem candidates. Finally the Viceroy asked Nehru to form the provisional government, which came into being on September 2, 1946. This great event, which caused Gandhi to refer to Nehru as "your uncrowned king and Prime Minister," was treated by Jinnah and the Moslem League as the signal for mourning and the display of black flags. There had been terrible Hindu-Moslem riots in Calcutta the month before, with at least five thousand killed and over fifteen thousand wounded; these were followed by outbreaks in a dozen different places in the new nation.

One of Gandhi's last great marches took place as a result of the inter-communal violence, which now, perhaps more than ever before, grieved him to the depths. He chose East Bengal for a long walk through the villages. He had been living in a hut in the untouchables' quarter in New Delhi, where members of the new government could consult him more or less at will. The outbreak of violence in East Bengal aroused him because it occurred in small villages, where, as a rule, Hindus and Moslems had always lived together without trouble. He decided to walk through the Noakhali and Tippera districts, where the murders had occurred, and see what he could do. He had not much hope; all this violence discouraged him and made him feel that his voice no longer had any power; but it was an inner necessity for him to try, even against the wishes of his old associates and the new government.

This journey across India was done in a special train, as had become usual and indeed necessary when the Mahatma traveled, for an ordinary train was so delayed that it upset the entire schedule. His special trains were made up of scrupulously clean third-class carriages. Enormous crowds gathered at every station, and the progress of such a train was necessarily erratic, but Gandhi got to Calcutta toward the end of October. New riots had broken out there just before, and were succeeded now by some terrible blood-lettings in the province of Bihar. Bihar was Hindu in the proportion of six to one, and the nationalist fanatics there proclaimed October 25 as "Noakhali Day" in revenge for the Moslem murders of Hindus in Noakhali. The dead were said to be over ten thousand in Bihar, mostly Moslems: thus each outrage brought forth a counter-outrage and each one worse than the other.

Gandhi at first thought of a fast as atonement for the Bihar massacre, but his original desire to go to East Bengal won out. He left Calcutta for Noakhali on November 7 and stayed in the district until March 2, 1947, walking from village to village. He wanted his immediate followers, women as well as men, to do the same, each living for a while in one village and attempting to quiet the angers and fears that had brought out violence. These were very poor villages of the delta country where the Ganges and the Brahmaputra run together, and there were neither roads nor transport. Gandhi himself stayed a few days in each village, sometimes no more than two days, and then walked on to the next, through country that had been cruelly hostile to Hindus, and with only three companions. For a large part of the time he walked barefoot. Sometimes the villages were half in ruins; there had been much looting; a good many frightened Hindus had gone away. The Mahatma kept on just the same, and the Mohammedans gathered by the thousand to listen to him. He preached his old message of brotherhood, purity of heart, forgive-ness for injuries. Before his pilgrimage was over, a very great improvement had taken place in the relations of Moslems and Hindus in the Noakhali and Tippera districts. He now departed to Bihar to carry the same message: "Everything I have to say is as old as the hills," he was wont to declare. In Bihar the Hindus were the wrongdoers and it was generally his way to be a little more severe with Hindus, his own people, than he ever was with Moslems. "I would forfeit my claim to being a Hindu," he said, "if I bolstered the wrongdoing of fellow-Hindus or of any other human being."

But while he was on this long journey of compassion, watched by all of India and a good part of the world, political affairs had reached a decisive phase. The Labour government was bent upon an immediate transfer of power in India, and for the first time named a date: "not later than June, 1948." In fact it took place on August 15, 1947. For the final negotiation and the actual transfer of power Mr. Attlee made an extremely auspi-cious choice as the last Viceroy: Admiral Lord Mount-batten, a man with the skill, charm, and intelligence required for the unparalleled task. He arrived in Delhi on March 22, 1947, and immediately invited Gandhi and Jinnah to come to the palace. Independence had, in fact, come: all that remained to be done was to fix its terms. It proved difficult indeed, and was accompanied and followed by dreadful disasters, but the thing itself was achieved at last. As Gandhi left Bihar for Delhi on what was to be the last of all his journeys, he must have thought that this was the end of a very long road, and in spite of all his sorrow, he must have had some pang of joy in the birth of freedom.

CHAPTER SEVEN

SACRIFICE AND FULFILLMENT

THE MAHATMA'S ordeal reached its most acute manifestations during the six or eight months before his assassination, mainly by the partition of India and the wave of human misery and physical misfortune that followed.

Gandhi got on well with Mountbatten, as did all Indian leaders. It was not Mountbatten's fault that the fundamental condition of Indian independence now seemed to be partition. Jinnah would accept nothing else, and Jinnah held one hundred million Moslems in the hollow of his hand. Mountbatten told him that he could have partition, but not at the price of taking vast numbers of Hindus and Sikhs into Pakistan against their will: a line of partition would have to be drawn that would cut right through the Punjab and right through Bengal, two provinces he had claimed in their entirety. Nehru, Rajaji, and the rest of the Congress leaders would accept this as the price of independence. Gandhi conceded their right to do so, as he conceded the existing fact of partition, but it never received his approval—never more than his passive acceptance. This (the acceptance) occurred at the prayer meeting in Delhi on June 4, 1947, and settled the fate of the British Empire.

But all through that awful summer and winter the Mahatma was in storm and travail. There were riots, murders, and bloodshed more or less everywhere. His influence had always been very strong with Moslems, his religious prestige with Hindus irresistible. He felt that nobody listened to him any more, that his life had been

wasted in an endeavor which came to no end, resulted
in no achievement. He wore himself out in a struggle to
make the people understand that they must love and
understand one another, forgive the past, and build a
future. Wherever he himself went, the message seemed
to be understood, because of the magical power of his
own gentle, pleading person, but he would then receive
telegraphed dispatches from other parts of the country
saying that his pleas for peace had been disregarded. The
Moslems were killing the Hindus and the Hindus were
killing the Moslems wherever the balance of numbers
made such massacres possible. It has been estimated that
several millions (as many as seven or eight) lost their
lives in this unprecedented mass murder, and something
like fifteen million people were uprooted from their
accustomed homes and hurled from Pakistan to India or
from India to Pakistan, seeking safety.

No greater suffering for Mahatma Gandhi could have
been invented or devised. This is what he had given his
life to prevent. He took his weary way again to Calcutta,
where mass violence had been prevalent, and there drove
or walked through the streets, talking to the people. He
got there six days before the transfer of power from
British to Indian hands. All his time he spent in an
endeavor to make Hindus and Moslems friendly to one
another. On the actual day of India's liberation, August
15, he passed his whole time in silence, fasting, and
prayer. The effect of his own presence was very great,
and there is small doubt that it restored peace to Calcutta,
which had been devastated by riots for a whole year.
But it was still not complete: the Mahatma fasted. This
time it was a "fast unto death" or until Calcutta had
returned to sanity. Within seventy-three hours Calcutta

had returned to sanity. And it remained sane: during all
the horrors of the next month or two in other parts of
India, peace remained in Calcutta. All the leaders of
both sides had promised the Mahatma to maintain the
peace, and they kept their word.

He left Calcutta on September 7 for Delhi, intending
to go to the Punjab, where the most serious violence of
all had broken out. He was implored to stay in Delhi
for the moment, at the government's wish.

He remained in Delhi, which was torn by evil-doing
of the most barbarous character. Between Delhi and the
Punjab he would spend his last efforts, sadly and wearily
and with death in his heart, but with the most unflagging
energy.

One of the greatest catastrophes in modern history,
perhaps in all history, was taking place. At one time
Gandhi said, in his evening prayer meeting: "It makes
my brain reel to think how this can be. Such a happening
is unparalleled in the history of the world, and it makes
me, as it should make you, hang my head in shame."

In Delhi itself, the capital of the new nation, murder
was rife. No street was safe. I arrived there on the heels
of the worst bloodshed and heard endless tales of it.
The Moslems had almost completely been driven out or
murdered by the time I got there. The Mahatma was
ceaselessly active, and wherever he went there was peace,
but he could not be everywhere at once. Hindus and
Sikhs were being murdered in Pakistan at the same time
and on the same scale. The Punjab was perhaps the worst
of all, and there the Mahatma wished to end his Indian
pilgrimage, as he had in one sense (at Amritsar) begun it.

It was not so to be. He began his last fast on January

13, 1948, for peace in Delhi itself. He felt that he could not go elsewhere so long as the capital was not safe for all citizens. "If Delhi goes, India goes, and with that the last hope of world peace," he said. He would fast unto death or until Delhi was at peace.

Those days were strange and solemn. The streets that had run with blood were filled with penitents of all ages, religions, and conditions, praying for the life of the Mahatma. Never shall I forget them. I spent much of my time reading Sophocles and talking to some of the Indian leaders. The fear of his death was prevalent everywhere, among foreigners as much as among Indians. In a sense, the whole country held its breath, and I have heard that essentially the same thing happened in Pakistan at the same moment.

The last fast ended with a pledge from all the principal leaders of Hinduism in Delhi and in India to keep the peace with their Moslem brethren. The Mahatma accepted a glass of orange juice from his old Moslem friend, the Maulana Sahib (January 18, 1948).

For twelve days Gandhi recuperated from his fast. He was carried to his evening prayer-meeting in a small, improvised wooden chair for the first few days, but thereafter walked in his sandals down the garden, leaning on "the girls" (his granddaughters or a granddaughter-in-law). Thus he walked on Friday, January 30, shortly after five in the afternoon. I was standing there waiting for him to come and noted by my watch that it was 5:12 when he appeared. This was unusually late, for he was due at five; and the official version says that he appeared at five past five. He mounted the few steps that led to the small terrace at the end of the garden, which he had appropriated as prayer-ground. Nathuram Vinayak

Godse, a young ultra-nationalist Hindu, bowed before
him, receiving his blessing, and then shot him dead.

2

The assassination of Gandhi was designed by its
perpetrator to remove an obstacle to war. It was thought
by Godse and his fellow conspirators that only Gandhi
was preventing war between India and Pakistan, a war
which, they considered, India would inevitably win, thus
reuniting the country by force.

What the assassin achieved was peace, not war. The
revulsion against war which swept over the entire sub-
continent was tremendous, and it was certainly sincere.
It was just as true in Pakistan as in India. In after weeks
I was on the Northwest Frontier itself, where the semi-
barbarous Pathans have no regard for peace. In certain
villages I was asked to describe how Gandhi died, and
I saw tears in some very tough eyes. The whole of India
and the whole of Pakistan mourned the apostle of peace,
and in so doing they brought about a psychological
condition in which war became totally impossible.

This may have preserved the peace of the world for
the duration of the present situation. Atomic energy
already had rendered war a horror to all informed men
of any imagination, but it had not yet been sufficiently
understood throughout the world. It needed another two
years, and perhaps three, to deliver its dreadful message.
If Pakistan and India had gone to war in 1948, as they
very obviously threatened to do, they might have dragged
the whole world into it before it had gone very far—
and indeed it is likely that this would have been the result.
The Mahatma's sacrifice was therefore a fulfillment. He
restored peace to "Delhi, India and the world," as he

had prayed. His death fulfilled his life, in the manner that has been the central characteristic of religious drama since the beginning of history. No less than Jesus of Nazareth, he died for all mankind. There could have been no better end for a life that was all devotion, all sacrifice, all abnegation and love. The man had no equal in our time, this one who treated all men as equals. Of all that we have known, he was the wisest and the best —as was said of Socrates in days of old.

BIBLIOGRAPHY

GANDHI's autobiography, under the title *My Experi-ments with Truth,* was published by the Navajivan Pub-lishing House at Ahmedabad, India. An edition issued by the Public Affairs Press in Washington, D.C., is the only American edition, and has been exhausted. This is the indispensable source for the story of his first forty-five years.

Louis Fischer's *Life of Mahatma Gandhi* (New York: Harper and Brothers, 1950) is probably the most fac-tual; my own *Lead, Kindly Light* (New York: Random House, 1949) is personal interpretation, as is Dr. John Haynes Holmes's *My Gandhi* (1953). *Mahatma Gan-dhi: His Own Story* (New York: The Macmillan Com-pany, 1930), edited by C. F. Andrews, consists of ex-cerpts from the autobiography and other works. The *Gandhi-Gita,* which is the *Gita* text translated by Maha-dev Desai and Gandhi, with the Gandhian interpretation, has never been published in the United States; it can be obtained from the Navajivan Publishing House.

Thoreau's essay on civil disobedience will be found in Volume IV of *The Writings of Henry David Tho-reau,* the 1906 edition.

Following is a partial list of books on Indian history, philosophy, or politics which might be found useful:

BESANT, ANNIE: *How India Wrought for Freedom* (*The Story of the National Congress Told from Of-ficial Records*). London: Theosophical Publishing House, 1915.

BEVAN, EDWYN: *Indian Nationalism.* New York: The Macmillan Company, 1914.

BHAGAVAN DAS: *The Science of the Self.* Benares: Indian Bookshop, 1938.

BLOOMFIELD, MAURICE: *The Religion of the Veda.* New York: G. P. Putnam's Sons, 1908.

CAVE, SYDNEY: *Redemption, Hindu and Christian.* New York: Oxford University Press, 1919.

The Cambridge History of India: Volume VI, *The Indian Empire.* London: Cambridge University Press, 1932.

CHAKRAVARTI, SURES CHANDRA: *The Philosophy of the Upanishads.* University of Calcutta, 1935.

CROOKE, W.: *The Popular Religion and Folklore of North India.* Two volumes. London: Constable & Co., 1896.

CUMMING, SIR JOHN (editor): *Political India, 1832–1932.* New York: Oxford University Press, 1932.

DUTT, R. PALME: *India Today.* London: Victor Gollancz, 1940.

ELIOT, SIR CHARLES: *Hinduism and Buddhism: An Historical Sketch.* Three volumes. New York: Longmans, Green & Company, 1921.

FARQUHAR, J. N.: *An Outline of the Religious Literature of India.* New York: Oxford University Press, 1920.

Gandhiji's Correspondence with the Government, 1942–1944. Ahmedabad: Navajivan Publishing House, 1945.

The Gita. Professor Radhakrishnan's translation is admirable, as is Christopher Isherwood's. Mrs. Besant's and Gandhi's are mentioned in this book. I like the one made by Shri Purohit Swami (a friend of William Butler Yeats, and influenced or helped by him), published in London in 1935 by Faber and Faber. Sir Edwin Arnold's *The Song Celestial* is the best-known metrical version.

MAJUMDAR, R. C., H. C. RAYCHAUDHURI, and KA-

LINKAR DATTA: *An Advanced History of India.* New York: The Macmillan Company, 1946.

MORELAND, W. H., and ATUL C. CHATTERJEE: *A Short History of India.* New York: Longmans, Green & Company, 1936.

MUZUMDAR, H. T.: *Gandhi Triumphant! The Inside Story of the Historic Fast.* New York: Universal Pub. Co., 1939.

OMAN, JOHN CAMPBELL: *Cults, Customs and Superstitions of India.* Philadelphia: G. W. Jacobs & Co., 1908.

RADHAKRISHNAN, S.: *Indian Philosophy.* Two volumes. London: George Allen and Unwin, 1931.

RAMAN, T. A.: *What Does Gandhi Want?* New York: Oxford University Press, 1942.

ROLLAND, ROMAIN: *Mahatma Gandhi.* Paris, 1924.

RAVOOF, A. A.: *Meet Mr. Jinnah.* Lahore: Sheikh Muhammad Ashraf, 1947.

SEN, GERTRUDE EMERSON: *Voiceless India.* Toronto: Longmans, Green & Company, 1946.

SHRIDHARANI, KRISHNALAL: *The Mahatma and the World.* New York: John Day Company, 1940.

SINGH, ANUP: *Nehru, the Rising Star of India.* New York: John Day Company, 1939.

SMITH, VINCENT: *The Oxford Student's History of India.* Revised by H. G. Rawlinson. New York: Oxford University Press, 1951.

SMITH, WILFRED CANTWELL: *Modern Islam in India.* London: Victor Gollancz, 1947.

SMITH, WILLIAM ROY: *Nationalism and Reform in India.* New Haven: Yale University Press, 1938.

SOCIALIST PARTY OF INDIA: *Policy Statement.* (By Jaiprakash Narayan.) Bombay: Socialist Party Central Office, 1947.

WHITEHEAD, HENRY: *The Village Gods of South India.* New York: Oxford University Press, 1921.

WOOLACOTT, J. E.: *India on Trial: A Study of Present Conditions*. New York: The Macmillan Company, 1929.

Anyone who wishes to go farther into Indian origins will find the standard German works—Oldenberg's *Buddha* and Paul Deussen's *Vedanta System of Philosophy*, for instance—well translated. Tagore's *Sadhana* (New York: The Macmillan Company, 1916) and some of the work of Shri Aurobindo, in particular his two volumes of *Essays on the Gita*, are valuable, but the latter can be obtained only from the Arya Publishing House, Calcutta. The Oxford University series called "The Religious Quest of India" contains a considerable number of enlightening works, some of which are named in the above list.

The files of *Young India* and of *Harijan* can be consulted only in India. A comprehensive edition of Gandhi's work is in preparation, but will take a long time to make ready.

INDEX

This book was set on the Linotype in a face called *El-dorado*, so named by its designer, WILLIAM ADDISON DWIGGINS, as an echo of Spanish adventures in the Western World. The series of experiments that culminated in this type-face began in 1942; the designer was trying a page more "brunette" than the usual book type. "One wanted a face that should be sturdy, and yet not too mechanical. . . . Another desideratum was that the face should be narrowish, compact, and close fitted, for reasons of economy of materials." The specimen that started Dwiggins on his way was a type design used by the Spanish printer A. de Sancha at Madrid about 1774. Eldorado, however, is in no direct way a copy of that letter, though it does reflect the Madrid specimen in the anatomy of its arches, curves, and junctions. Of special interest in the lower-case letters are the stresses of color in the blunt, sturdy serifs, subtly counterbalanced by the emphatic weight of some of the terminal curves and finials. The roman capitals are relatively open, and winged with liberal serifs and an occasional festive touch.

This book was composed by The Plimpton Press, Norwood, Massachusetts, and printed and bound by The Book Press, Brattleboro, Vt. The typography and binding were designed by the creator of its type-face— W. A. Dwiggins.